# Medical Spanish
## made ridiculously simple

**Trudy Espinoza-Abrams**
How to Examine a Spanish-Speaking Patient
Without Knowing a *Single* Word of Spanish

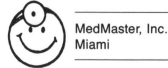

MedMaster, Inc.
Miami

*Made in the United States of America*

Published by
MedMaster, Inc.
P.O. Box 640028
Miami, FL 33164


ISBN 0-940780-45-3

## DEDICATION

To Dick, Jessina and Erin.

*Todo es posible*

# PREFACE

For many years I thought of writing a book to help Hispanic patients make themselves understood to English-speaking health-care personnel. First as an undergraduate and graduate training programs coordinator in a medical school department of psychiatry, and later as an advisor in the Dean for Students' office, I encountered many residents and medical students asking for my assistance in translating medical terms to help them communicate with their patients. It was during these years that I appreciated the real need for a book such as this.

I have written the book so that someone who doesn't speak or understand a word of Spanish can pick it up and elicit all the necessary medical information from an exclusively Spanish-speaking patient. Its three-column organization: *English, Spanish* and *Phonetic Spanish*, makes it simple to use. The medical questions are short and direct, to facilitate phonetic pronunciation, and are phrased to elicit only *"Yes"* or *"No"* answers, so that the examiner without any comprehension of Spanish can immediately understand the answers to all questions.

The text follows the standard medical interview format as presented in Swartz' <u>Physical Diagnosis</u>, so that any health-care professional can interview a patient by simply following a familiar outline. The *Index of Common Symptoms and Signs* allows the interviewer to rapidly find the specific questions he needs, without having to thumb through the entire book. The *Dictionary of Medical Terminology*, and the companion *Glossary of Medical Terms in Spanish*, further enhance the ease of using this volume.

With Hispanics now constituting the largest U.S. minority population, health care professionals who don't speak or understand Spanish are increasingly faced with often-insurmountable interviewing difficulties when, as is more and more frequently the case, bilingual interpreters with a knowledge of medical terminology are unavailable. It is my hope that the present volume will help to fill this gap, and thereby increase the quality of care offered and received.

Trudy Espinoza-Abrams
*Vernon Hills, Illinois*
*April, 1992*

## ACKNOWLEDGEMENT

It is with sincere appreciation that I thank my husband, Richard Abrams, M.D., for his invaluable contribution to the making of this book; without his help, encouragement and support, it would not have been possible to complete it.

## ABOUT THE AUTHOR

Trudy Espinoza-Abrams worked for many years at University of Health Sciences/The Chicago Medical school, first in the doctoral program in Clinical Psychology, then as Programs Coordinator for the undergraduate and graduate training programs in the Department of Psychiatry and Behavioral Sciences, and eventually in the office of the Dean for Students, where her experience counseling medical students ultimately led her to write this book.

Born and raised in Granada, Nicaragua, Mrs. Espinoza-Abrams immigrated to the U.S. in her teens, graduating high school in Miami and obtaining her college degree during a tour of duty in the Navy. She now makes her home in Vernon Hills, Illinois, with her physician husband and two teen-age daughters.

# TABLE OF CONTENTS

## Greetings and General Remarks

| | | |
|---|---|---|
| *Hello* | Hola, Halo | **Oh**-lah, Ah-**low** |
| *Good Morning* | Buenos Días | **Bweh**-nohs **Dee**-ahs |
| *Good Afternoon* | Buenas Tardes | **Bweh**-nahs **Tahr**-dehs |
| *Good Evening/Night.* | Buenas Noches | **Bweh**-nahs **Noh**-chehs |
| *Morning* | Mañana | Mah-**nyah**-nah |
| *Afternoon* | Tarde | **Tahr**-deh |
| *Evening/Night* | Noche | **Noh**-cheh |
| *Have a:* | Que pase: | Keh **Pah**-seh: |
| * good evening | Buenas Noches | **Bweh**-nahs **Noh**-chehs |
| * good day | Buen Día | Bwehn **Dee**-ah |
| * good afternoon | Buenas tardes | **Bweh**-nahs **tahr**-dehs |
| *I am Jane Doe, a doctor (student) in this hospital.* | Yo soy Jane Doe, un(a) doctor(a) (estudiante) en este hospital. | Joh soy (as in soy beans) **Jah**-neh Doh-**eh**, oon(a) **duck**-tohr(ah) (ehs-too-**dee-ahn**-teh) ehn **ehs**-teh ohs-pee-**tahl**. |
| *How are you? (polite)* | Como esta usted? | **Koh**-moh ehs-**tah** oos-**tehd**? |
| *How are you? (informal)* | Que Tal? | Keh **tahl**? |
| *How is it going?* | Como le va? | **Koh**-moh leh **vah**? |
| *Mr.; Sir* | Señor | Seh-**nyohr** |
| *Mrs.; Mistress* | Señora | Seh-**nyoh**-rah |
| *Miss* | Señorita | Seh-nyoh-**ree**-tah |
| *I need to ask you a few questions.* | Necesito hacerle unas preguntas. | Neh-seh-**see**-toh ah-**sehr**-leh **ooh**-nahs preh-**goon**-tahs. |
| *When answering, please speak slowly.* | Cuándo conteste, por favor hable despacio. | **Kwahn**-doh kohn-**tehs**-teh, pohr fah-**vohr ah**-bleh dehs-**pah**-see-oh. |
| *I speak only a little Spanish.* | Hablo sólo un poquito de Español. | **Ah**-bloh **soh**-loh oon poh-**kee**-toh deh Ehs-pah-**nyohl**. |

| Answer "yes" or "no" to the following questions: | Conteste "si" o "no" a las siguientes preguntas: | Kohn-**tehs**-teh "see" oh "noh" ah lahs see-**gee-ehn**-tehs preh-**goon**-tahs: |
|---|---|---|
| Do you speak English? | Habla Inglés? | **Ah**-blah Een-**glehs**? |
| Is there anyone with you who speaks English? | Hay alguién con usted que hable Inglés? | Eye ahl-**gee-ehn** kohn oos-**tehd** keh **ah**-bleh Een-**glehs**? |
| What is your: | Cual es su: | Kwahl ehs soo: |
| * first name? | * primer nombre? | * pree-**mehr** **nohm**-breh? |
| * last name? | * apellido? | * ah-peh-**yee**-doh? |
| What _____ were you born? | En que _____ nació usted? | Ehn keh _____ nah-**see-oh** oos-**tehd**? |
| * month | * mes | * mehs |
| * date | * día | * **dee**-ah |
| * year | * año | * **ah**-nyoh |
| Are you presently: | Es usted : | Ehs oos-**tehd**: |
| * single (male)? (female) | * soltero? (soltera?) | * sol-**teh**-roh? (sol-**teh**-rah?) |
| * married? | * casado? (casada?) | * kah-**sah**-doh? (kah-**sah**-dah?) |
| * divorced? | * divorciado? (divorciada?) | * dee-vohr-**see-ah**-doh? (dee-vohr-**see-ah**-dah?) |
| * widowed? | * viudo? (viuda?) | * vee-**oo**-doh? (vee-**oo**-dah?) |
| What is your: | Cual es su: | Kwahl ehs soo: |
| * address? | * dirección? | * dee-reg-**see-ohn**? |
| * city? | * ciudad? | * see-oo-dahd? |
| * phone number? | * número de teléfono? | * **noo**-meh-roh deh teh-**leh**-foh-noh? |
| Whom do we notify of your stay here? | A quién notificamos de su estadía aquí? | Ah kee-**ehn** noh-tee-fee-**kah**-mohs deh soo ehs-tah-**dee**-ah ah-**kee**? |
| Do you have any children? | Tiene hijos? (hijas?) | **Tee-eh**-neh ee-hohs? (**ee**-hahs?) |

2

| Show me with your fingers how many. | Enséñeme con sus dedos cuántos. | Ehn-**seh**-nyeh-meh kohn soos **deh**-dohs **kwahn**-tohs. |
| Are you employed? | Está usted empleado? | Ehs-**tah** oos-**tehd** ehm-pleh-**ah**-doh? |
| Do you have health insurance? | Tiene usted seguro de hospitalización? | **Tee-eh**-neh oos-**tehd** seh-**goo**-roh deh **ohs**-pee-tah-lee-sah-**see-ohn**? |
| What is the name of your insurance company? | Cual es el nombre de su compañia de seguro? | Kwahl ehs ehl **nohm**-breh deh soo kohm-pah-**nyee-ah** deh seh-**goo**-roh? |
| Do you carry an insurance card with you? | Lleva consigo la tarjeta de seguro? | **Jeh**-vah kohn-**see**-goh lah tahr-**heh**-tah deh seh-**goo**-roh? |
| May I see the card? | Puedo ver la tarjeta? | **Pweh**-doh vehr lah tahr-**heh**-tah? |
| This form authorizes us to check you this hospital. | Este formulario nos autoriza admitirlo en este hospital. | **Ehs**-teh fohr-moo-**lah**-ree-oh nohs outoh-**ree**-in sah ad-mee-**teer**-loh ehn **ehs**- teh ohs-**pee**-tahl. |
| Please, sign here. | Por favor, firme aqui. | Pohr fah-**vohr**, **feer**-meh ah-**kee**. |

## Present Illness

| Have you been ill long? | Ha estado enfermo por mucho tiempo? | Ah ehs-**tah**-doh ehn-**fehr**-moh pohr **moo**-choh **tee-ehm**-poh? |
| Are you having any: | Tiene usted alguna de: | **Tee-eh**-neh oos-**tehd** ahl-**goo**-nah deh: |
| Have you had any of these before now: | Ha tenido uno de estos antes: | Ah teh-**nee**-doh **oo**-noh deh **ehs**-tohs **ahn**-tehs: |
| * bleeding? | * desangre? | * deh-**sahn**-greh? |
| * cough? | * tos? | * tohs? |
| * diarrhea? | * diarrea? | * dee-ah-**rheh-ah**? |
| * dizzy spells? | * mareos? | * mah-**reh**-ohs? |
| * fever? | * fiebre? | * **fee-eh**-breh? |
| * pain? | * dolor? | * doh-**lohr**? |
| * problem breathing? | * problema al respirar? | * proh-**bleh**-mah ahl rehs-pee-**rahr**? |

| English | Spanish | Pronunciation |
|---|---|---|
| * vomiting? | * vomitos? | * **voh**-mee-tohs? |
| Did you last have any of the above: | Tuvo alguno de lo mencionado: | **Too**-voh ahl-**goo**-noh deh loh **mehn**-see-oh-**nah**-doh: |
| * day before yesterday? | * El dia antes de ayer? | * Ehl **dee-ah** ahn-tehs deh ah-**yhehr**? |
| * last month? | * el mes pasado? | * ehl mehs pah-**sah**-doh? |
| * last night? | * anoche? | * ah-**noh**-cheh? |
| * last week? | * la semana pasada? | * lah seh-**mah**-nah pah-**sah**-dah? |
| * two days ago? | * dos dias atras? | * dohs **dee**-ahs ah-**trahs**? |
| * yesterday? | * ayer? | * ah-**yhehr**? |
| Did (the pain) it just start again? | Acaba de empezar el dolor otra vez? | Ah-**kah**-bah deh ehm-peh-**sahr** ehl doh-**lohr** **oh**-trah vehs? |
| How many hours (days, weeks, months) has it been this way? | Cuántas horas (dias, semanas, meces) hace de dolerle? | **Kwahn**-tahs **oh**-rahs (**dee**-ahs) seh-**mah**-nahs, **meh**-ses) **ah**-seh deh doh-**lehr**-leh? |
| Please count on your fingers | Por favor cuente en sus dedos | Pohr fah-**vohr kwehn**-teh ehn soos **deh**-dohs. |
| Is (the pain) it worse at some times and not others? | Es el dolor peor unas veces que otras? | Ehs ehl doh-**lohr** peh-**ohr oo**-nahs **veh**-sehs keh oh-**trahs**? |
| Is (the pain) it steady? | Es el dolor continuo? | Ehs ehl doh-**lohr** kohn-**tee**-nwoh? |
| Does (the pain) it change? | Cambia de intensidad? | **Kahm**-bee-ah deh een-**tehn**-see-dahd? |
| Does (the pain) it affect your perforwork? | Le afecta el dolor en su trabajo? | Leh ah-**feh**-tah ehl doh-**lohr** ehn **soo** mance at trah-**bah**-hoh? |
| Point with your finger where it hurts the most. | Señale con un dedo donde le duele mas. | Seh-**nyah**-leh kon oon **deh**-doh **dohn**-deh leh **dweh**-leh mahs. |
| Does the pain spread to other parts? | Se extiende el dolor a otras partes? | Seh egs-**tee-ehn**-deh ehl doh-**lohr** ah **oh**-trahs **pahr**-tehs? |

| Show me from where to where. | Enséñeme de donde a donde. | Ehn-**seh**-nyeh-meh d **dohn**-deh ah **dohn**-d |
|---|---|---|
| *Is the pain:* | Es el dolor: | Ehs ehl doh-**lohr**: |
| * aching? | * doloroso? | * doh-loh-**roh**-soh? |
| * burning? | * ardiente? | * ahr-dee-**ehn**-teh? |
| * constant? | * constante? | * kohns-**tahn**-teh? |
| * cramping? | * retortijante (retorcijante)? | * reh-tohr-**tee**-hahn-teh (reh-tohr-**see**-hahn-teh)? |
| * dull? | * monótono? | * moh-**noh**-toh-noh? |
| * intermittent? | * intermitente? | * een-**tehr**-mee-**tehn**-teh? |
| * mild? | * ligero? | * lee-**heh**-roh? |
| * moderate? | * moderado? | * moh-deh-**rah**-doh? |
| * severe? | * severo? | * seh-**veh**-roh? |
| * sharp? | * afilado? | * ah-fee-**lah**-doh? |
| * squeezing? | * apretante? | * ah-preh-**tahn**-teh? |
| * throbbing? | * pulsante? | * pool-**sahn**-teh? |
| *Does it make you:* | El dolor le da: | Ehl doh-**lohr** leh dah: |
| * dizzy? | * mareos? | * mah-**reh**-ohs? |
| * have insomnia? | * insomnia? | * een-**some**-nee-ah? |
| * lose your appetite? | * falta de apetito? | * **fahl**-tah deh ah-peh-**tee**-toh? |
| * nauseous? | * náuseas? | * **nah**-oo-seahs? |
| *Do you get the pain:* | Le da a usted el dolor: | Leh dah ah oos-**tehd** ehl doh-**lohr**: |
| * after meals? | * después de comer? | * dehs-**pwehs** deh koh-**mehr**? |
| * before meals? | * antes de comer? | * **ahn**-tehs deh koh-**mehr**? |
| *Is the pain worse when:* | Es peor el dolor cuando: | Ehs peh-**ohr** ehl doh-**lohr** **kwahn**-doh: |
| * breathing? | * respira? | * rehs-**pee**-rah? |
| * exerting | * hace esfuerzo por | * **ah**-seh ehs-**fwehr**-soh |

| | | |
|---|---|---|
| yourself? | sí mismo? | pohr **see mees**-moh? |
| * moving your bowels? | * pasando el excremento? | * pah-**sahn**-doh ehl egs-kreh-**mehn**-toh? |
| * urinating? | * orina? | * oh-**ree**-nah? |
| *Does the pain awaken you from sleep?* | Lo despierta el dolor cuando duerme? | Loh dehs-**pee-ehr**-tah ehl doh-**lohr kwahn**-doh **dwehr**-meh? |
| *Have you taken any medication for the pain?* | Ha tomado alguna medicina para el dolor? | Ah toh-**mah**-doh ahl-**goo**-nah meh-dee-**see**-nah **pah**-rah el doh-**lohr**? |
| *Did this medication help you?* | Le ayudó la medicina? | Leh ah-you-**doh** lah meh-dee-**see**-nah? |
| *Do you have the bottle with you?* | Tiene la botella con usted? | **Tee-eh**-neh lah boh-**teh**-yah kohn oos-**tehd**? |
| *Please show me the bottle.* | Por favor enséñeme la botella. | Pohr fah-**vohr** ehn-**seh**-nyeh-meh lah boh-**teh**-yah. |
| *Does heat (cold) make it feel better?* | Lo hace sentir mejor una bolsa caliente (de hielo)? | Loh **ah**-seh sehn-**teer** meh-**hohr oo**-nah **bohl**-sah-kah-**lee-ehn**-teh (deh **yeh**-loh)? |
| *Does any phlegm (sputum) come up?* | Tiene flema en la garganta? | **Tee-eh**-neh **fleh**-mah ehn lah gahr-**gahn**-tah? |
| *Is the phlegm:* | Es la flema: | Ehs lah **fleh**-mah: |
| * yellow? | * amarilla? | * ah-mah-**ree**-yah? |
| * white? | * blanca? | * **blahn**-kah? |
| * clear? | * clara? | * **klah**-rah? |
| * green? | * verde? | * **vehr**-deh? |
| * grey? | * gris? | * grees? |
| *How much phlegm per day do you get:* | Cuánto de flema obtiene al dia: | **Kwahn**-toh deh **fleh**-mah ob-**tee-eh**-neh ahl **dee**-ah: |
| * one teaspoon? | * una cucharadita? | * **oo**-nah **koo**-chah-rah-**dee**-tah? |
| * one tablespoon? | * una cucharada? | * **oo**-nah koo-chah-**rah**-dah? |
| * 1/2 a cup? | * media taza? | * **meh**-dee-ah **tah**-sah? |

6

| | | |
|---|---|---|
| Do you get the coughing attack: | Le coge el ataque de tos: | Leh **koh**-heh ehl ah-**tah**-keh deh tohs: |
| * in the daytime? | * durante el dia? | * doo-**rahn**-teh ehl **dee**-ah? |
| * at nighttime? | * durante la noche? | * doo-**rahn**-teh lah **noh**-cheh? |
| Does sitting up (lying) down make it better? | El sentarse (acostarse) le hace sentir mejor? | Ehl sehn-**tahr**-seh (ah-kohs-**tahr**-seh) leh **ah**-seh sehn-**teer** meh-**horh**? |
| Does anything make it feel better? Worse? | Hay algo que lo hace sentir mejor? Peor? | Eye **ahl**-goh keh loh **ah**-seh sehn-**teer** meh-**hohr**? **Peh**-ohr? |
| Have you coughed up blood? | Ha tocido sangre? | Ah toh-**see**-doh **sahn**-greh? |
| Do you smoke cigarettes? | Fuma cigarrillos? | **Foo**-mah see-gah-**rhee**-yohs? |
| How many per day? | Cuántos al dia? | **Kwahn**-tohs ahl **dee**-ah? |
| Before this illness, have you been in good health? | Antes de esta enfermedad ha tenido buena salud? | **Ahn**-tehs deh **ehs**-tah ehn-fehr-meh-dad ah teh-**nee**-doh **bweh**-nah sah-**lood**? |
| Have your symptoms kept you in bed? | Lo han mantenido en cama los sintomas? | Loh ahn mahn-teh-**nee**-doh ehn **kah**-mah lohs **seen**-toh-mahs? |
| Have you been getting better? worse? | Se ha mejorado? empeorado? | Seh ah ▪**meh**-hoh-**rah**-doh **ehm**-peh-oh-**rah**-doh? |
| Have you been in an accident? | Ha estado en un accidente? | Ah ehs-**tah**-doh ehn oon agsee-**dehn**-teh? |
| Please, show me your injury. | Por favor, enséñeme donde se dañó. | Pohr fah-**vohr** ehn-**seh**-nyeh-meh **dohn**-deh seh dah-**nyoh**. |

## Past History

Past Illness/Family History:

| | | |
|---|---|---|
| Have you ever had: Have any of your relatives had: | Ha tenido usted: Alguno de sus parientes ha tenido: | Ah teh-**nee**-doh oos-**tehd**: Ahl-**goo**-noh deh soos pah-**ree**-**ehn**-tehs ah teh-**nee**-doh: |

| English | Spanish | Pronunciation |
|---|---|---|
| * allergies? | * alergias? | * ah-**lehr**-hee-ahs? |
| * anemia? | * anemia? | * ah-**neh**-mee-ah? |
| * arthritis? | * artritis? | * are-**treeh**-tees? |
| * asthma? | * asma? | * **ahs**-mah? |
| * cancer? | * cancer? | * **kahn**-sehr? |
| * chicken pox? | * viruela (varicela)? | * vee-**rweh**-lah (vah-ree-**seh**-lah)? |
| * measles? | * sarampión? | * sah-rahm-**pee-ohn**? |
| * mumps? | * paperas? | * pah-**peh**-rahs? |
| * congenital abnormalities? | * anormalidades congenitas? | * ah-nohr-mah-lee-**dah**-dehs kohn-**heh**-nee-tahs? |
| * diabetes? | * diabetes? | * dee-ah-**beh**-tehs? |
| * emphysema? | * enfisema? | * ehn-fee-**seh**-mah? |
| * epilepsy? | * epilepsia? | * eh-pee-**lep**-see-ah? |
| * heart disease? | * enfermedad del corazón? | * **ehn**-fehr-meh-dad dehl koh-rah-**sohn**? |
| * hepatitis? | * hepatitis? | * **eh**-pah-**tee**-tees? |
| * high blood pressure? | * presión alta? | * preh-**see-ohn** ahl-tah? |
| * mental disease? | * enfermedad mental? | * **ehn**-fehr-meh-dad mehn-**tahl**? |
| * rheumatic fever? | * fiebre reumática? | * **fee-eh**-breh reh-oo-**mah**-tee-kah? |
| * stroke? | * derrame? | * deh-**rhah**-meh? |
| * syphilis? | * sífilis? | * **see**-fee-lees? |
| * tuberculosis? | * tuberculosis? | * too-**behr**-koo-**loh**-sees? |
| * ulcers? | * ulceras? | * **ool**-seh-rahs? |
| *Were you exposed to:* | Fue expuesto a: | **Fweh** egs-**pwehs**-toh ah: |
| * an infection? | * una infección? | * **oo**-nah een-feg-**see-ohn**? |
| * a contagious illness? | * una enfermedad contagiosa? | * **oo**-nah **ehn**-fehr-meh-dad kohn-tah-**hee-oh**-sah? |

## Allergies:

| | | |
|---|---|---|
| *Have you had:* | Ha tenido usted: | Ah teh-**nee**-doh oos-**tehd**: |
| * a history of asthma or chronic bronchitis? | * historial de asma o bronquitis crónica? | * ees-toh-**ree**-**ahl** deh **ahs**-mah oh brohn-**kee**-tees **kroh**-nee-kah? |
| * a sudden coughing attack while eating? | * un ataque súbito de tos mientras come? | * oon ah-**tah**-keh **soo**-bee-toh deh tohs **mee**-**ehn**-trahs **koh**-meh? |
| * hives/urticaria? | * urticarias? | * oor-tee-**kah**-ree-ahs? |
| *Have you:* *Has the patient had:* | Ha usted: Ha el paciente: | Ah oos-**tehd**: Ah ehl pah-**see**-**ehn**-teh: |
| * been exercising or exerting himself? | * estado ejercitando o esforzandose? | * ehs-**tah**-doh eh-**her**-see-**tahn**-doh-seh oh ehs-fohr-**sahn**-doh-seh? |
| * been exposed to allergens? | * sido expuesto a alérgenes? | * **see**-doh egs-**pwehs**-toh ah ah-**lehr**-heh-nehs? |
| * developed unexplained wheezing or coughing? | * adquirido inexplicable respiración silbante o tos? | * adkee-**ree**-doh eenegs-plee-**kah**-bleh rehs-**pee**-rah-**see**-**ohn** seel-**bahn**-teh oh tohs? |
| * had a recent respiratory infection? | * tenido una infeccion respiratoria reciente? | * teh-**nee**-doh **oo**-nah een-feg-**see**-**ohn** rehs-pee-rah-**toh**-ree-ah reh-**see**-**ehn**-teh? |
| * had a strong emotional stress? | * tenido mucha tension emocional? | * teh-**nee**-doh **moo**-chah tehn-**see**-**ohn** eh-moh-see-oh-**nahl**? |
| * had a family history of asthma? | * tenido historial de asma en la familia? | * teh-**nee**-doh ees-toh-**ree**-**ahl** deh **ahs**-mah ehn lah fah-**mee**-lee-ah? |

## Hospitalization: Injury/Surgery:

| | | |
|---|---|---|
| *Have you been in a hospital before?* | Ha estado en el hospital antes? | Ah ehs-**tah**-doh ehn ehl ohs-**pee**-tahl **ahn**-tehs? |
| *Did you have:* | Tuvo usted: | **Too**-voh oos-**tehd**: |
| * surgery? | * una operación? | * **oo**-nah **oh**-peh-rah-**see**-**ohn**? |

9

| * a serious injury? | * un accidente (daño) serio? | * oon agsee-**dehn**-teh (**dah**-nyoh) **seh**-ree-oh? |
|---|---|---|
| *Show me where the* operation (injury) was. | Enséñeme donde fue la operación (daño serio). | Ehn-**seh**-nyeh-meh **dohn**-deh **fweh** lah oh-peh-rah-**see-ohn** (**dah**-nyoh **seh**-ree-oh). |
| *Did you have the* surgery/serious injury a long time ago or recently? | Tuvo la operación/daño serio hace tiempo o recientemente? | **Too**-voh lah oh-peh-rah-**see-ohn** ah-seh **tee-ehm**-poh oh reh-**see-ehn**-teh-mehn-teh? |
| *Have you ever had:* | Ha tenido usted: | Ah teh-**nee**-doh oos-**tehd**: |
| * any broken bones? | * huesos quebrados? | * **weh**-sohs keh-**brah**-dohs? |
| * a head injury? | * un daño a la cabeza? | * oon **dah**-nyoh ah lah kah-**beh**-sah? |
| * concussion? | * concusiones cerebrales? | * kohn-koo-**see-oh**-nehs **seh**-reh-brah-lehs? |
| *Have you ever been* unconscious? | Ha perdido el conoci-miento alguna vez? | Ah pehr-**dee**-doh ehl koh-noh-see-**mee-ehn**-toh ahl-**goo**-nah vehs? |

Medication:

| *Do you take any of the* following: | Toma alguno de los siguiente: | **Toh**-mah ahl-**goo**-noh deh lohs see-**gee-ehn**-teh: |
|---|---|---|
| * antacids? | * antiácidos? | * **ahn**-tee-**ah**-see-dohs? |
| * antibiotics? | * antibióticos? | * **ahn**-tee-**bee-oh**-tee-kohs? |
| * anticoagulants? | * anticoagulantes? | * **ahn**-tee-koh-ah-goo-**lahn**-tehs? |
| * anticonvulsants? | * anticonvulsantes? | * **ahn**-tee-kohn-vool-**sahn**-tehs? |
| * blood pressure medications? | * medicina para presión alta? | * meh-dee-**see**-nah **pah**-rah preh-**see-ohn** **ahl**-tah? |
| * diet pills? | * pastillas de dieta? | * pahs-**tee**-yhahs deh **dee-eh**-tahs? |
| * heart pills? | * pastillas del corazón? | * pahs-**tee**-yhahs dehl koh-rah-**sohn**? |

10

| | | |
|---|---|---|
| * laxatives? | * laxantes? | * lag-**sahn**-tehs? |
| * narcotics? | * narcóticos? | * nahr-**koh**-tee-kohs? |
| * pain killers? | * pastillas para dolor? | * pahs-**tee**-yhahs **pah**-rah doh-**lohr**? |
| * sedatives? | * sedativos? | * seh-dah-**tee**-vohs? |
| * tranquillizers? | * tranquilizantes? | * trahn-kee-lee-**sahn**-tehs? |
| * vitamins? | * vitaminas? | * vee-tah-**mee**-nahs? |
| * any (other) kind of medication? | * otra clase de medicina? | * **oh**-trah **klah**-seh deh meh-dee-**see**-nah? |
| *Do you have the bottle with you?* | Tiene la botella con usted? | **Tee-eh**-neh lah boh-**teh**-yah kohn oos-**tehd**? |
| *Please show me the bottle.* | Por favor enséñeme la botella. | Pohr fah-**vohr** ehn-**seh**-nyeh-meh lah boh-**teh**-yah. |
| *Are you allergic to any medication?* | Es alérgico a alguna medicina? | Eh ah-**lehr**-hee-koh ah ahl-**goo**-nah meh-dee-**see**-nah? |
| *Are you allergic to:* | Es usted alérgico a la: | Ehs oos-**tehd** ah-**lehr**-hee-koh ah lah: |
| * penicillin? | * penicilina? | * peh-nee-see-**lee**-nah? |
| * other kinds of medication? | * otra clase de medicina? | * **oh**-trah **klah**-seh deh meh-dee-**see**-nah? |
| * bee or hornet stings? | * picadura de abeja o avispón? | * pee-kah-**doo**-rah deh ah-**beh**-hah oh ah-vees-**pohn**? |

Drugs:

| | | |
|---|---|---|
| *Do you use drugs?* | Usa usted drogas? | **Oo**-sah oos-**tehd droh**-gahs? |
| *Do you use any drugs to make you feel better?* | Usa alguna droga para sentirse mejor? | **Oo**-sah ahl-**goo**-nah **droh**-gah **pah**-rah sehn-**teer**-seh meh-**hohr**? |
| *Which of the following do you use:* | Cuál de los siguiente usa usted: | Kwahl deh lohs see-gee-**ehn**-teh **oo**-sah oos-**tehd**: |
| * amphetamines/speed? | * anfetaminas? | * ahn-feh-tah-**mee**-nahs? |
| * Angel dust or PCP? | * Polvo de | * **Pohl**-voh deh **ahn**-hehl |

| English | Spanish | Pronunciation |
|---|---|---|
| | ángel o PCP? | oh Peh-Seh-Peh? |
| * barbiturates? | * barbitúricos (diablos)? | * bahr-bee-**too**-ree-kohs (dee-ah-blohs)? |
| * cocaine or crack? | * cocaina (coca)? | * koh-kah-**ee**-nah (**koh**-kah)? |
| * downers? | * abajos (depresantes)? | * ah-**bah**-hohs (deh-preh-**sahn**-tehs)? |
| * heroin? | * heroina? | * eh-roh-**ee**-nah? |
| * uppers? | * estimulantes? | * ehs-tee-moo-**lahn**-tehs? |
| *Do you use them daily?* | Los usa a diario? | Lohs **oo**-sah ah **dee-ah**-ree-oh? |
| *Do you ever share needles with others?* | Ha compartido jeringas con otros? | Ah kohm-pahr-**tee**-doh heh-**reen**-gas kohn **oh**-trohs? |
| *Have you ever been arrested on drug charges?* | Ha sido arrestado alguna vez por drogas? | Ah **see**-doh ah-**rhehs**-tah-doh ahl-**goo**-nah vehs pohr **droh**-gahs? |
| *Have you ever over-dosed on drugs?* | Se ha sobre drogado alguna vez? | Seh ah soh-breh droh-**gah**-doh ahl-**goo**-nah vehs? |
| *When was your last drug dose?* | Cuando fué su ultima dosis? | **Kwahn**-doh **fweh** soo **ool**-tee-mah **doh**-sees? |
| *Have you been through a detoxification-program?* | Ha participado en un programa de desintoxicación? | Ah pahr-**tee**-see-**pah**-doh ehn oon proh-**grah**-mah deh deh-seen-tog-see-fee-kah-**see**-**ohn**? |
| *Have you ever taken methadone for detoxing?* | Ha tomado metadona para desintoxicarse? | Ah toh-**mah**-doh meh-tah-**doh**-nah **pah**-rah deh-seen-**tog**-see-kahr-seh? |
| *Have you ever gotten yellow jaundice or hepatitis?* | Alguna ves le ha dado hepatitis o ictericia amarilla? | Ahl-**goo**-nah vehs leh ah **dah**-doh eh-pah-**tee**-tees oh eeg-teh-**ree**-see-ah ah-mah-**ree**-yah? |
| *Have you checked your blood for AIDS?* | Se ha hecho el examen de sangre para el SIDA? | Seh ah **eh**-choh ehl eg-**sah**-mehn deh **sahn**-greh **pah**-rah ehl **See**-dah? |
| *Has the use of drugs or alcohol ever caused you problems with:* | El uso de drogas o alcohol le ha causado problemas con: | Ehl **oo**-soh deh **droh**-gahs oh ahl-**kohl** leh ah kah-oo-**sah**-doh proh-**bleh**-mahs kohn: |

12

| | | |
|---|---|---|
| * your family? | * su familia? | * soo fah-**mee**-lee-ah? |
| * the law? | * las leyes? | * lahs **leh**-yhehs? |
| * your finances? | * sus financias? | * soos fee-**nahn**-see-ahs? |
| * your health? | * su salud? | * soo sah-**lood**? |
| * your job? | * su trabajo? | * soo trah-**bah**-hoh? |
| * your friends? | * sus amigos? | * soos ah-**mee**-gohs? |

| | | |
|---|---|---|
| *Have you ever sought help for your:* | Ha buscado ayuda por su: | Ah boos-**kah**-doh ah-**you**-dah pohr soo: |
| * drinking problem? | * problema con el licor? | * proh-**bleh**-mah kohn ehl lee-**kohr**? |
| * drug usage? | * uso de drogas? | * **oo**-soh deh **droh**-gahs? |

Alcohol:

| | | |
|---|---|---|
| *Do you drink alcohol?* | Toma usted alcohol (licor)? | **Toh**-mah oos-**tehd** ahl-**kohl** (lee-**kohr**)? |
| *Do you drink:* | Toma usted: | **Toh**-mah oos-**tehd**: |
| * beer? | * cerveza? | * sehr-**veh**-sah? |
| * wine? | * vino? | * **vee**-noh? |
| * hard liquor? | * licor fuerte? | * lee-**kohr** **fwehr**-teh? |
| *How many drinks/beers do you drink daily?* | Cuántos tragos o cervezas se toma diario? | **Kwahn**-tohs **trah**-gohs oh ser-**veh**-sahs seh **toh**-mah **dee-ah**-ree-oh? |
| *Do you drink :* | Toma alcohol: | **Toh**-mah ahl-**kohl**: |
| * every day? | * cada día? | * **kah**-dah **dee**-ah? |
| * before breakfast? | * antes del desayuno? | * **ahn**-tehs dehl **deh**-sah-**you**-noh? |
| * at work? | * en el trabajo? | * ehn ehl trah-**bah**-hoh? |
| *Have you started drinking recently?* | Ha empezado a tomar recientemente? | Ah ehm-peh-**sah**-doh ah toh-**mahr** reh-**see-ehn**-teh-mehn-teh? |
| *Have you been drinking for years now?* | Ya ha tomado licor por años? | Yah ah toh-**mah**-doh lee-**kohr** pohr **ah**-nyohs? |
| *Have you ever:* | Ha usted: | Ah oos-**tehd**: |

| | | |
|---|---|---|
| * been arrested for driving while intoxicated? | * sido arrestado por manejar intoxicado? | * **see**-doh ah-rhehs-**tah**-doh por mah-neh-**hahr** een-**tog**-see-**kah**-doh? |
| * attended a meeting of Alcoholics Anonymous? | * atendido una reunión de Alcoholicos Anónimos? | * ah-tehn-**dee**-doh **oo**-nah reh-oo-**nee-ohn** deh Ahl-**koh**-lee-kohs Ah-**noh**-nee-mohs? |
| * had the Delirium Tremens? | * tenido trémulos de delirio? | * teh-**nee**-doh **treh**-moo-lohs deh deh-**lee**-ree-oh? |
| * missed work because of drinking? | * perdido trabajo por el tomar? | * pehr-**dee**-doh trah-**bah**-hoh pohr ehl toh-**mahr**? |
| * had blackouts for what happened while you were drinking? | * perdido la memoria de lo que pasa cuando toma? | * pehr-**dee**-doh lah meh-**moh**-ree-ah deh loh keh **pah**-sah **kwahn**-doh **toh**-mah? |

Immunizations:

| | | |
|---|---|---|
| *Are you up to date on your immunizations?* | Está al día con sus vacunas? | Ehs-**tah** ahl **dee**-ah kohn soos vah-**koo**-nahs? |
| *Do you know what immunizations you need?* | Sabe que vacunas necesita? | **Sah**-beh keh vah-**koo**-nahs neh-seh-**see**-tah? |
| *Do you know when was the last time you had a tetanus shot?* | Sabe cuando fue la última ves que tuvo la vacuna del tétano? | **Sah**-beh **kwahn**-doh fweh lah ool-**tee**-mah vehs keh **too**-voh lah vah-**koo**-nah dehl **teh**-tah-noh? |
| *Has it been more than ten years?* | Hace mas de dies años? | **Ah**-seh mahs deh dee-**ehs** ah-**nyohs**? |
| *You should have a tetanus shot now.* | Debe de tener la vacuna del tétano ahora. | **Deh**-beh deh teh-**nehr** lah vah-**koo**-nah dehl **teh**-tah-noh ah-**oh**-rah. |

Travel:

| | | |
|---|---|---|
| *Have you recently travelled to a foreign country?* | Ha viajado a otro pais recientemente? | Ah vee-ah-**hah**-doh ah **oh**-troh pah-**ees** reh-see-**ehn**-teh-mehn-teh? |
| *Which country?* | Que pais? | Keh pah-**ees**? |
| *Did you drink any of their water?* | Bebió del agua de alli? | Beh-**bee-oh** dehl ah-gwah deh ah-yee? |
| *Did you only drink bottled water?* | Tomó sólo agua en botella? | Toh-**moh soh**-loh **ah**-gwah ehn boh-**teh**-yhah? |

| English | Spanish | Pronunciation |
|---|---|---|
| *Did you use any ice?* | Usó hielo? | Oo-**soh** **yeh**-loh? |
| *Did you eat any fruits with their skins?* | Comió alguna fruta con cascara? | Koh-**mee-oh** ahl-**goo**-nah **froo**-tah kohn **kahs**-kah-rah? |

Occupational History:

| English | Spanish | Pronunciation |
|---|---|---|
| *Do you work?* | Trabaja usted? | Trah-**bah**-hah oos-**tehd**? |
| *Where do you work?* | En donde trabaja? | Ehn **dohn**-deh trah-**bah**-hah? |
| *What kind of work do you do?* | Que clase de trabajo hace? | Keh **klah**-seh deh trah-**bah**-hoh **ah**-seh? |
| *Have you been here long?* | Ha estado alli por mucho tiempo? | Ah ehs-**tah**-doh ah-**yee** pohr **moo**-choh **tee-ehm**-poh? |
| *At work, are you exposed to:* | En el trabajo esta expuesto a: | Ehn ehl trah-**bah**-hoh ehs-**tah**- egs-**pwehs**-toh ah: |
| * dusts? | * polvos? | * **pohl**-vohs? |
| * fumes? | * gases? | * **gah**-sehs? |
| * chemical solvents? | * soluciones quimicas? | * soh-loo-**see-oh**-nehs kee-mee-kahs? |
| * other hazardous material? | * otras materias peligrosas? | * **oh**-trahs mah-**teh**-ree-ahs peh-lee-**groh**-sahs? |
| *Do you use protective clothing or equipment?* | Usa ropa o equipo protectores? | **Oo**-sah **roh**-pah oh eh-**kee**-poh proh-**teg**-toh-rehs? |
| *Do you wear a mask?* | Usa mascara? | **Oo**-sah **mahs**-kah-rah? |
| *Does anyone in your household work with hazardous materials?* | Alguien en su familia trabaja con materias peligrosas? | Ahl-**gee-ehn** ehn soo fah-**mee**-lee-ah trah-**bah**-hah kohn mah-**teh**-ree-ahs peh-lee-**groh**-sahs? |
| *Have you ever lived close to a:* | Alguna vez ha vivido cerca de un: | Ahl-**goo**-nah vehs ah vee-**vee**-doh **sehr**-kah deh oon: |
| * chemical laboratories? | * laboratorio quimico? | * lah-boh-rah-**toh**-ree-oh **kee**-mee-koh? |
| * nuclear waste facilities? | * basurero nuclear? | * **bah**-soo-**reh**-roh noo-kleh-**ahr**? |
| * other hazardous facilities? | * otras facilidades dañinas? | * **oh**-trahs fah-see-lee-**dah**-dehs dah-**nyee**-nahs? |

15

| | | |
|---|---|---|
| *Have you lost time from work?* | Ha perdido días de trabajo? | Ah pehr-**dee**-doh **dee**-ahs deh trah-**bah**-hoh? |
| Was it due to the kind of job you do? | Los perdió a causa del trabajo que hace? | Lohs pehr-**dee**-oh ah kah-**oo**-sah dehl trah-bah-hoh keh **ah**-seh? |

Psychosocial history:

| | | |
|---|---|---|
| *Have you noticed any:* | Ha notado algun: | Ah noh-**tah**-doh ahl-**goon**: |
| * mood swings lately? | * cambio de humor ultimamente? | * **kahm**-bee-oh deh oo-**moh ool**-tee-mah-**mehn**-teh? |
| * weight loss? | * perdida de peso? | * **pehr**-dee-dah deh **peh**-soh? |
| * palpitations? | * palpitaciones? | * **pahl**-pee-tah-**see-oh**-nehs? |
| *Do you feel:* | Se siente usted: | Seh **see-ehn**-teh oos-**tehd** |
| * confused? | * confundido? | * kohn-foon-**dee**-doh? |
| * depressed? | * deprimido? | * deh-pree-**mee**-doh? |
| * nervous? | * nervioso? | * nehr-**vee-oh**-soh? |
| * restless? | * intranquilo? | * een-trahn-**kee**-loh? |
| * shaky? | * tembloroso? | * tehm-bloh-**roh**-soh? |
| * weak? | * debil? | * **deh**-beel? |
| *Do you have any of the following:* | Tiene algo de los siguientes: | **Tee-eh**-neh **ahl**-goh deh lohs see-**gee-ehn**-tehs: |
| * anxiety? | * ansiedad? | * **ahn**-see-eh-dad? |
| * depression? | * depresión? | * **deh**-preh-**see-ohn**? |
| * insomnia? | * insomnia? | * een-**some**-nee-ah? |
| * loss of appetite? | * perdida de apetito? | * **pehr**-dee-dah deh ah-peh-**tee**-toh? |
| * loss of interest? | * perdida de interés? | * **pehr**-dee-dah deh een-teh-**rehs**? |
| * memory loss? | * perdida de memoria? | * **pehr**-dee-dah deh meh-**moh**-ree-ah? |
| * thoughts of death or suicide? | * pensamientos de muerte o suicidio? | * pehn-sah-**mee-ehn**-tohs deh mwehr-teh oh swee-**see**-dee-oh? |

| Do you want to hurt: | Quiere lastimar: | **Kee-eh**-reh lahs-tee-mahr |
|---|---|---|
| * yourself? | * asi mismo? | * ah-**see mees**-moh? |
| * others? | * a otros? | * ah **oh**-trohs? |
| Do you want to die? | Quiere morirse? | **Kee-eh**-reh moh-**reer**-seh? |
| Have you recently lost a family member? | Se le ha muerto un familiar reciente-mente? | Seh leh ah **mwehr**-toh oon fah-mee-**lee-ahr** reh-**see-ehn**-teh-**mehn**-teh? |
| A loved one? | Un ser querido? | Oon sehr keh-**ree**-doh? |
| Do you sleep well at night? | Duerme bien en las noches? | **Dwehr**-meh bee-**ehn** ehn lahs **noh**-chehs? |
| Are you satisfied with your sexual performance? | Esta satisfecho con su forma sexual? | Ehs-**tah** sah-**tees**-feh-choh kohn soo **fohr**-ma **seg**-swal? |
| Do you think your partner is satisfied? | Cree que su compañero esta satisfecho? | Kreh-**eh** keh soo kohm-pah **nyeh**-roh ehs-**tah** sah-tees-**feh**-choh? |
| Do you want to talk about your sex life? | Quiere hablar acerca de su vida sexual? | **Kee-eh**-reh ah-**blahr** ah-**sehr**-kah deh soo **vee**-dah seg-swal? |
| Do you have any pro-blems achieving an orgasm? | Tiene problemas en lograr un orgasmo? | **Tee-eh**-neh proh-**bleh**-mahs ehn loh-**grahr** oon ohr-**gas**-moh? |
| Have you ever felt disappointment in your sexual functions? | Se ha sentido decep-cionado en su funcion sexual? | Seh ah sehn-**tee**-doh deh **sep**-see-oh-**nah**-doh ehn soo foon-**see-ohn** seg-swal? |
| How often do you have intercourse: | Cada cuánto hace el amor: | **Kah**-dah **kwahn**-toh **ah**-seh ehl ah-**mohr**: |
| * every day? | * cada dia? | * **kah**-kah **dee**-ah? |
| * twice a day? | * dos veces al dia? | * dohs **veh**-sehs ahl **dee**-ah? |
| * three days a week? | * tres dias a la semana? | * trehs **dee**-ahs ah lah seh-**mah**-nah? |
| * once a week? | * una vez a la semana? | * **oo**-nah vehs ah lah seh-**mah**-nah? |
| * once a month? | * una vez al mes? | * **oo**-nah vehs ahl mehs? |

17

| English | Spanish | Pronunciation |
|---|---|---|
| *Do you try new positions and activities?* | Prueba nueva posiciones y actividades? | **Prweh**-bah **nweh**-vah poh-see-**see**-**oh**-nehs ee ag-tee-vee**dah**-dehs? |
| *Do you get an erection and maintain it throughout?* | Obtiene una erección y la mantiene hasta el final? | Ob-**tee**-**eh**-neh **oo**-nah eh-reg-**see**-**ohn** ee lah mahn-**tee**-**eh**-neh **ahs**-tah ehl fee-**nahl**? |

Diet:

| English | Spanish | Pronunciation |
|---|---|---|
| *Do you remember what you ate yesterday for:* | Se acuerda que comió ayer en el: | Seh ah-**kwehr**-dah keh koh-**mee**-**oh** ah-**yher** ehn ehl: |
| * breakfast? | * desayuno? | * **deh**-sah-**you**-noh? |
| * lunch? | * almuerzo? | * ahl-**mwehr**-soh? |
| * dinner? | * cena? | * **seh**-nah? |
| * snacks? | * meriendas? | * meh-**ree**-**ehn**-dahs? |
| *Do you snack when watching t.v.?* | Come meriendas cuando ve la t.v.? | **Koh**-meh meh-**ree**-**ehn**-dahs **kwahn**-doh veh lah teh-veh? |
| *How many times a week do you eat:* | Cuantas veces en la semana come: | **Kwahn**-tahs **veh**-sehs ehn lah seh-**mah**-nah **koh**-meh: |
| * meat? | * carne? | * **kahr**-neh? |
| * fish? | * pescado? | * pehs-**kah**-doh? |
| * chicken or turkey? | * pollo o pavo? | * **poh**-yhoh oh **pah**-voh? |
| *Do you eat lots of:* | Come mucho: | **Koh**-meh **moo**-choh: |
| * green salads? | * ensaladas verde? | * **ehn**-sah-**lah**-dahs **vehr**-deh? |
| * broccoli? | * bróculi? | * **broh**-koo-lee? |
| * carrots? | * zanahorias? | * **sah**-nah-**oh**-ree-ahs? |
| * other vegetables? | * otros vegetales? | * **oh**-trohs veh-**heh**-tah-lehs? |
| * whole grain breads? | * pan de granos? | * pahn deh **grah**-nohs? |
| * bran cereals? | * cereal de afrecho? | * seh-**reh**-**ahl** deh ah-**freh**-choh? |
| * other high fiber | * otras comidas altas | * **oh**-trahs koh-**mee**-dahs |

| | | |
|---|---|---|
| * fresh fruits? | * frutas frescas? | * **froo**-tahs **frehs**-kahs? |
| * salt? | * sal? | * sahl? |
| * fried/spicy foods? | * comidas fritas/ picantes? | * koh-**mee**-dahs **free**-tahs/ pee-**kahn**-tehs? |
| *Do you have a food intolerance?* | Tiene alguna intole- rancia a comidas? | **Tee-eh**-neh ahl-**goo**-nah **een**toh-leh-**rahn**-see-ah ah koh-**mee**-dahs? |
| *How many cups of tea or coffee do you drink daily?* | Cuantas tazas de té o café toma diario? | **Kwahn**-tahs **tah**-sahs deh **teh** oh kah-**feh** **toh**-mah dee-**ah**-ree-oh? |
| *How often do you eat chocolate:* | Cada cuánto come chocolate: | **Kah**-dah **kwahn**-toh **koh**-meh choh-koh-**lah**-teh: |
| * everyday? | * cada día? | * **kah**-dah **dee**-ah? |
| * every other day? | * cada otro día? | * **kah**-dah **oh**-troh **dee**-ah? |
| * once a week? | * una vez a la semana? | * **oo**-nah vehs ah lah seh-**mah**-nah? |
| *Do you do any kind of exercise?* | Hace alguna clase de ejercicios? | * **Ah**-seh ahl-**goo**-nah **klah**-seh deh eh-hehr- **see**-see-ohs? |
| *Do you exercise by:* | Hace ejercicios: | **Ah**-seh eh-hehr-**see**- see-ohs: |
| * running? | * corriendo? | * koh-**ree-ehn**-doh? |
| * walking? | * caminando? | * kah-mee-**nahn**-doh? |
| * dancing? | * bailando? | * bah-ee-**lahn**-doh? |
| * aerobics? | * de aerobios? | * deh ah-eh-**roh**-bee-ohs? |
| * swimming? | * nadando? | * nah-**dahn**-doh? |
| * weight lifting? | * levantando pesas? | * leh-vahn-**tahn**-doh **peh**-sahs? |
| *Do you exercise for:* | Hace ejercicio por: | **Ah**-seh eh-hehr-**see**- see-ohs pohr: |
| * less than half an hour a day? | * menos de media hora al día? | * **meh**-nohs deh **meh**-dee- ah **oh**-rah ahl **dee**-ah? |
| * more than half an hour a day? | * mas de media hora al día? | * mahs deh **meh**-dee-ah **oh**-rah ahl **dee**-ah? |

| At what time do you go to sleep? | A que hora se acuesta a dormir? | Ah keh **oh**-rah seh ah-**kwehs**-tah ah **dohr**-meehr? |
| Do you have any problems falling asleep? | Tiene problemas en dormirse? | **Tee-eh**-neh proh-**bleh**-mahs ehn dohr-**meer**-seh? |
| Do you sleep the night through? | Se duerme la noche completa? | Seh **dwehr**-meh lah **noh**-cheh kohm-**pleh**-tah? |
| Do you awaken in the middle of the night? | Se despierta en medio de la noche? | Seh dehs-**pee-ehr**-tah ehn **meh**-dee-oh deh lah **noh**-cheh? |
| Do you have trouble falling back to sleep? | Tiene problemas en dormirse nuevamente? | **Tee-eh**-neh proh-**bleh**-mahs ehn dohr-**meer**-seh **nweh**-vah-mehn-teh? |

## Review of Systems/Physical Examination

### General:

| Have you noticed any of the following: | Ha notado uno de los siguientes: | Ah noh-**tah**-doh **oo**-noh deh lohs see-**gee-ehn**-tehs: |
| * chills? | * escalofrios? | * ehs-kah-loh-**free-ohs**? |
| * fatigue? | * fatiga? | * fah-**tee**-gah? |
| * fever? | * fiebre? | * **fee-eh**-breh? |
| * irritability? | * irritabilidad? | * **eer**hee-tah-bee-lee-dad? |
| * night sweats? | * sudor de noche? | * soo-**dohr** deh **noh**-cheh? |
| * paralysis? | * parálisis? | * pah-**rah**-lee-sees? |
| * weakness? | * debilidad? | * **deh**-beeh-lee-**dad**? |
| Show me how high the fever was. | Enséñeme que alta fué la fiebre. | Ehn-**seh**-nyeh-meh keh **ahl**-tah **fweh** lah **fee-eh**-breh. |
| (Ask patient/parent to point to thermometer) | | |
| Have you gained any weight lately? | Ha subido de peso últimamente? | Ah soo-**bee**-doh deh **peh**-soh **ool**-tee-mah-**mehn**-teh? |
| Have you experienced tiredness? | Ha sentido mucho cansancio? | Ah sehn-**tee**-doh **moo**-choh kahn-**sahn**-see-oh? |
| Do you feel tired: | Se siente cansado: | Seh **see-ehn**-teh kahn-**sah**-doh: |
| * all day long? | * todo el día? | * **toh**-doh ehl **dee**-ah? |

| * in the morning? | * en la mañana? | * ehn lah mah-**nyah**-nah? |
|---|---|---|
| * in the evening? | * en la noche? | * ehn lah **noh**-cheh? |
| *Do you feel less tired in the morning?* | Se siente menos cansado en la mañana? | Seh **see-ehn**-teh **meh**-nohs kahn-**sah**-doh ehn lah mah-**nyah**-nah? |
| *Do you feel more tired at:* | Se siente mas cansado en: | Seh **see-ehn**-teh mahs kahn-**sah**-doh ehn: |
| * home? | * casa? | * **kah**-sah? |
| * work? | * el trabajo? | * ehl trah-**bah**-hoh? |
| *Is the fatigue relieved by rest?* | Se le mejora la fatiga con descanso? | Seh leh meh-**hoh**-rah lah fah-**tee**-gah kohn dehs-**kahn**-soh? |
| *Do you have weakness in your arms or legs?* | Tiene debilidad en sus brazos o pies? | **Tee-eh**-neh **deh**-bee-lee-dad ehn soos **brah**-sohs oh pee-ehs? |
| *You are now going to have a physical examination.* | Ahora le voy a dar un examen físico. | Ah-**oh**-rah leh voy ah dahr oon eg-**sah**-mehn **fee**-see-koh. |
| *Please relax.* | Por favor, relajese. | Pohr fah-**vohr** reh-lah-**heh**-seh. |
| *Take off your clothes and put this gown on.* | Quítese la ropa y póngase este camizón. | **Kee**-teh-seh lah **rhoh**-pah ee **pohn**-gah-seh **ehs**-teh kah-mee-**sohn**. |
| *Do you generally feel well?* | Generalmente se siente bien? | **Heh**-neh-rahl-**mehn**-teh seh **see-eh**-teh bee-ehn? |
| *Do you have problems with your hearing or vision?* | Tiene problemas con sus oídos o vista? | **Tee-eh**-neh pro-**bleh**-mahs kohn soos oh-**ee**-dohs oh **vees**-tah? |
| *Do you have trouble smelling or tasting things properly?* | Tiene problemas al oler o probar cosas? | **Tee-eh**-neh proh-**bleh**-mahs ahl oh-**lehr** oh proh-**bahr** **koh**-sahs? |

Blood Pressure:

| *Let me take your blood pressure.* | Dejeme tomarle la presión. | **Deh**-heh-meh toh-**mahr**-leh lah preh-**see-ohn**. |
|---|---|---|
| *Your blood pressure is normal.* | Su presión es normal. | Soo preh-**see-ohn** ehs nohr-**mahl**. |
| *Your blood pressure* | Su presión está | Soo preh-**see-ohn** ehs-**tah** |

21

| is high. | alta. | **ahl**-tah. |
| *Your blood pressure is low.* | Su presión está baja. | Soo preh-**see-ohn** ehs-tah **bah**-hah. |

## Pulse:

| *I need to take your pulse.* | Necesito tomarle el pulso. | Neh-seh-**see**-toh toh-**mahr**-leh ehl **pool**-soh. |
| *Your pulse is too rapid.* | Su pulso es muy rápido. | Soo **pool**-soh ehs mooy **rah**-pee-doh. |
| *Your pulse is too slow.* | Su pulso es muy lento. | Soo **pool**-soh ehs mooy **lehn**-toh. |
| *Your pulse is irregular.* | Su pulso es irregular. | Soo **pool**-soh ehs ee-rheh-goo-**lahr**. |
| *Your pulse is normal.* | Su pulso es normal. | Soo **pool**-soh ehs nohr-**mahl**. |

## Temperature:

| *I am going to take your temperature.* | Voy a tomarle su temperatura. | Voy ah toh-**mahr**-leh soo tehm-peh-rah-**too**-rah. |
| *You have a high fever.* | Tiene fiebre (calentura) alta. | **Tee-eh**-neh **fee-eh**-breh (kah-lehn-**too**-rah) **ahl**-tah. |
| *You have a slight fever.* | Tiene un poco de fiebre (calentura). | **Tee-eh**-neh oon **poh**-koh deh **fee-eh**-breh (kah-lehn-**too**-rah). |

## Skin:

| *Have you had the rash for long?* | Hace tiempo que tiene el salpullido? | **Ah**-seh **tee-ehm**-poh keh **tee-eh**-neh ehl sahl-poo-**yee**-doh? |
| *Have you ever had:* | Ha tenido alguna vez: | Ah teh-**nee**-doh ahl-**goo**-nah vehs: |
| * abnormal pigmentation? | * manchas anormales en la piel? | * mahn-**chahs** ah-nohr-**mah**-lehs ehn lah pee-ehl? |
| * eczema? | * eccema? | * egg-**seh**-mah? |
| * hives? | * urticarias? | * oor-tee-**kah**-ree-ahs? |
| * jaundice? | * ictericia (piel amarilla)? | * eeg-teh-**ree**-see-ah (pee-ehl ah-mah-**ree**-yhah)? |

| * rash? | * salpullido? | * sahl-poo-**yee**-doh? |
|---|---|---|
| * skin disease? | * enfermedad de la piel? | * **ehn**-fehr-meh-**dad** deh lah pee-ehl? |
| *Have you had any change in the dryness of your skin?* | Ha tenido algún cambio en la sequedad de su piel? | Ah teh-**nee**-doh ahl-**goon kahm**-bee-oh ehn lah seh-keh-**dad** deh soo pee-ehl? |
| *Did the itching start suddenly?* | Le empezó la comezón de pronto? | Leh ehm-peh-**soh** lah koh-meh-**sohn** deh **prohn**-toh? |
| *Was the itching associated with a rash?* | Le empezó la picazón con salpullido? | Leh ehm-peh-**soh** lah pee-kah-**sohn** kohn sahl-poo-**yee**-doh? |
| *Did the rash begin:* | Empezó el salpullido: | Ehm-peh-**soh** ehl sal-poo-**yee**-doh: |
| * flat? | * plano? | * **plah**-noh? |
| * blistered? | * con ampollas? | * kohn ahm-**poh**-yahs? |
| *Is the lesion:* | Esta la lesión: | Ehs-**tah** lah leh-**see**-**ohn**: |
| * tender? | * delicada? | * deh-lee-**kah**-dah? |
| * numb? | * entumecida? | * ehn-too-meh-**see**-dah? |
| * burning? | * ardiente? | * ahr-**dee**-**ehn**-teh? |
| * itching? | * con comezón? | * kohn koh-meh-**sohn**? |
| *Have there been new lesions?* | Han habido nuevas lesiones? | Ahn ah-**bee**-doh **nweh**-vahs leh-**see**-**oh**-nehs? |
| *Was the rash caused by the sun?* | Fue causado el salpullido por el sol? | Fweh kah-oo-**sah**-doh ehl sahl-poo-**yee**doh pohr ehl sohl? |
| *Have you the rash on your body?* | Tiene el salpullido en el cuerpo? | **Tee-eh**-neh ehl sahl-poo-**yee**-doh ehn ehl **kwehr**-poh? |
| *Has there been anyone in your family with a similar rash?* | Ha habido alguien en su familia con el mismo salpullido? | Ah ah-**bee**-doh ahl-**gee**-**ehn** ehn soo fah-**mee**-lee-ah kohn ehl **mees**-moh sahl-poo-**yee**-doh? |
| *Have you been in close contact with that person?* | Ha tenido mucho contacto con esa persona? | Ah teh-**nee**-doh **moo**-choh kohn-**tag**-toh kohn **eh**-sah pehr-**soh**-nah? |
| *Do you have a history* | Tiene historial de | **Tee-eh**-neh ees-**toh**-ree- |

23

| | | |
|---|---|---|
| of allergy? | alergias? | ahl deh ah-**lehr**-hee-ahs? |
| *Have you loss any of your hair?* | Ha perdido algo de su pelo? | Ah pehr-**dee**-doh ahl-goh deh soo peh-loh? |
| *Has your hair loss occurred suddenly?* | La perdida de pelo ocurrió de repente? | Lah **pehr**-dee-dah deh **peh**-loh oh-koo-**ree-oh** deh rheh-**pehn**-teh? |
| *Has the change in hair loss been associated with:* | El cambio en su pelo esta asociado con: | Ehl **kahm**-bee-oh ehn soo **peh**-loh **ehs**-tah ah-soh-**see-ah**-doh kohn: |
| * fever? | * fiebre? | * **fee-eh**-breh? |
| * itching? | * comezón? | * koh-meh-**sohn**? |
| * recent stress? | * reciente tensión? | * reh-**see-ehn**-teh tehn-**see-ohn**? |
| * rash? | * salpullido? | * sahl-poo-**yee**-doh? |
| *Have you noticed any nail changes recently?* | Ha notado un cambio reciente en las uñas? | Ah noh-**tah**-doh oon **kahm**-bee-oh reh-**see-ehn**-teh ehn lahs **oo**-nyahs? |
| *Are you exposed to chemicals at home or work?* | Está expuesto a sustancias químicas en la casa o trabajo? | Ehs-**tah** egs-**pwehs**-toh ah soos-**tahn**-see-ahs **kee**-mee-kahs ehn lah **kah**-sah oh trah-**bah**-hoh? |
| *Do you ____ easily?* | Usted _____ con facilidad? | Oos-**tehd** _____ kohn fah-see-lee-**dad**? |
| * bruise | * magulla | * mah-**goo**-yah |
| * bleed | * sangra | * **sanh**-grah |

Head:

| | | |
|---|---|---|
| *Have you suffered from a:* | Ha sufrido de un: | Ah soo-**free**-doh deh oon: |
| * head injury? | * daño a la cabeza? | * **dah**-nyoh ah lah kah-**beh**-sah? |
| * head trauma? | * trauma a la cabeza? | * **trah**-oo-mah ah lah kah-**beh**-sah? |
| * trauma? | * trauma? | * **trah**-oo-mah? |
| *Do you get:* | Le cogen a usted: | Leh **koh**-hen ah oos-**tehd**: |
| * dizzy spells? | * mareos? | * mah-**reh**-ohs? |

| | | |
|---|---|---|
| * vomiting? | * vomitos? | * **voh**-mee-tohs? |
| * headache over your eyes? | * dolor de cabeza sobre sus ojos? | * doh-**lohr** deh kah-**beh**-sah **soh**-breh soos **oh**-hos? |
| * headaches? | * dolores de cabeza? | * doh-**loh**-rehs deh kah-**beh**-sah? |
| * spots before your eyes? | * manchas enfrente de sus ojos? | * **mahn**-chahs ehn-**frehn**-teh deh soos **oh**-hohs? |
| *Is the pain:* | Siente el dolor: | **See-ehn**-teh ehl doh-**lohr**: |
| * all over? | * por todos lados? | * pohr **toh**-dohs **lah**-dohs? |
| * behind one eye? | * atras de un ojo? | * ah-**trahs** deh oon **oh**-hoh? |
| * just over the temple? | * sólo en la sién? | * **soh**-loh ehn lah see-**ehn**? |
| * like a tightness? | * como un apretamiento? | * **koh**-moh oon ah-**preh**-tah-**mee-ehn**-toh? |
| * only on one side? | * sólo en un lado? | * **soh**-loh ehn oon **lah**-doh? |
| * worst in the back of your neck? | * peor en su nuca? | * peh-**ohr** ehn soo **noo**-kah? |
| *Does it awaken you from sleep?* | Lo despierta el dolor cuando duerme? | Loh dehs-**pee-ehr**-tah ehl doh-**lohr kwahn**-doh **dwehr**-meh? |
| *Is the skin or scalp tender?* | Se le pone la piel o cabellera adoloridas? | Seh leh **poh**-nehn lah pee-ehl oh kah-beh-**yheh**-rah ah-doh-loh-**ree**-dahs? |
| *Do the headaches come in groups?* | Los dolores de cabeza vienen en grupos? | Lohs doh-**loh**-rehs deh kah-**beh**-sah **vee-eh**-nehn ehn **groo**-pohs? |
| *Are you sensitive to:* | Es sensitivo a la: | Ehs sehn-see-**tee**-voh ah lah: |
| * light? | * luz? | * loos? |
| * noises? | * ruidos? | * **rwee**-dohs? |
| *Does it help to:* | Le ayuda cuando: | Leh ah-**you**-dah **kwahn**-doh: |
| * close your eyes? | * cierra los ojos? | * **see-eh**-rhah lohs **oh**-hohs? |

25

| | | |
|---|---|---|
| * sleep? | * duerme? | * **dwehr**-meh? |
| * apply pressure? | * aplica presión? | * ah-**plee**-kah preh-**see-ohn**? |
| * apply cold? | * aplica la bolsa de hielo? | * ah-**plee**-kah lah **bohl**-sah deh **yeh**-loh? |
| Does it last for: | Le dura por: | Leh **doo**-rah pohr: |
| * minutes? | * minutos? | * mee-**noó**-tohs? |
| * hours? | * horas? | * **oh**-rahs? |
| * days? | * días? | * **dee**-ahs? |
| Does Aspirin help? | Le ayuda la Aspirina? | Leh ah-**you**-dah lah Ahs-pee-**ree**-nah? |
| Do you suffer from | Sufre usted de: | **Soo**-freh oos-**tehd** deh: |
| * dizziness? | * mareos? | * mah-**reh**-ohs? |
| * fainting or fainting spells? | * desmayos o desvanecimientos? | * des-**mah**-yohs oh **dehs**-vah-neh-see-**mee-ehn**-tohs? |
| * fainting only when first standing up? | * desmayos cuando se para o levanta? | * dehs-**mah**-yohs **kwahn**-doh seh **pah**-rah oh leh-**vahn**-tah? |
| * fainting after urinating? | * desmayos despues de orinar? | * dehs-**mah**-yohs dehs-**pwehs** deh oh-**ree**-nahr? |
| * migraines? | * migrañas? | * mee-**grah**-nyahs? |
| Were you unsteady while walking? | Se sintió tambaleante al caminar? | Seh seen-**tee-oh** tahm-bah-**leh-ahn**-teh ahl kah-mee-**nahr**? |
| Did you feel like the room was spinning? | Sintió como si el cuarto daba vueltas? | Seen-**tee-oh koh**-moh see ehl **kwahr**-toh **dah**-bah **vwehl**-tahs? |
| Did you experience any nausea or vomiting during the attack? | Tuvo nauseas o vomitos durante el ataque? | **Too**-voh **nah**-oo-seh-ahs oh **voh**-mee-tohs doo-**rahn**-teh ehl ah-**tah**-keh? |
| Do you have any problem with your ears? | Tiene algun problema con sus oidos? | **Tee-eh**-neh ahl-**goon** proh-**bleh**-mah kohn soos oh-**ee**-dohs? |
| Do you get ringing in the ears? | Le coge zumbido en sus oidos? | Leh **koh**-heh soom-**bee**-doh ehn soos oh-**ee**-dohs? |

26

| Is the dizziness worse with your eyes open/ closed? | Es peor el mareo con sus ojos abiertos/ cerrados? | Ehs peh-**ohr** ehl mah-**reh**-oh kohn soos **oh**-hohs ah-**bee-ehr**-tohs/ seh-**rah**-dohs? |

Eyes:

| Follow my finger with your eyes. | Siga mi dedo con sus ojos. | **See**-gah mee **deh**-doh kohn soos **oh**-hohs. |
| Look at this light and follow it with your eyes. | Mire ésta luz y sígala con sus ojos. | **Mee**-reh **ehs**-tah loos ee **see**-gah-lah kohn soos **oh**-hos. |
| Let me feel your neck. | Déjeme sentir su nuca. | **Deh**-heh-meh sehn-**teer** soo **noo**-kah. |
| Look up. | Mire hacia arriba. | **Mee**-reh **ah**-see-ah ah-**ree**-bah. |
| Look down. | Mire hacia abajo. | **Mee**-reh **ah**-see-ah ah-**bah**-hoh. |
| Look here. | Mire aquí. | **Mee**-reh ah-**kee**. |
| Look right. | Mire a la derecha. | **Mee**-reh ah lah deh-**reh**-chah. |
| Look left. | Mire a la izquierda. | **Mee**-reh ah la ees-**kee-ehr**-dah. |
| Now look at my nose, please. | Ahora mire a mi nariz, por favor. | Ah-**oh**-rah **mee**-reh ah mee nah-**rees**, pohr fah-**vohr**. |
| How many fingers do you see? | Cuántos dedos vé usted? | **Kwahn**-tohs **deh**-dohs veh oos-**tehd**? |
| Do you ever have: | Ha tenido usted: | Ah teh-**nee**-doh oos-**tehd**: |
| * spots before your eyes? | * manchas enfrente de sus ojos? | * **mahn**-chahs ehn-**frehn**-teh deh soos **oh**-hohs? |
| * blurred vision? | * su vista nublada? | * soo **vees**-tah noo-**blah**-dah? |
| * double vision? | * doble visión? | * **doh**-bleh vee-**see-ohn**? |
| Did the loss of vision occur suddenly? | La pérdida de su vista ocurrió de repente? | Lah **pehr**-dee-dah deh soo **vees**-tah oh-koo-ree-**oh** deh reh-**pehn**-teh? |
| Does light bother you | Le molesta la luz? | Leh moh-**lehs**-tah lah loos? |
| Do you have pain when | Le dá dolor el | Leh dah doh-**lohr** ehl |

27

| blinking? | parpadear? | **pahr**-pah-deh-ahr? |
|---|---|---|
| *Is the pain:* | Es el dolor: | Ehs ehl doh-**lohr**: |
| * aching? | * doloroso? | * doh-loh-**roh**-soh? |
| * burning? | * ardiente? | * ahr-**dee-ehn**-teh? |
| * constant? | * constante? | * kohns-**tahn**-teh? |
| * dull? | * monótono? | * moh-**noh**-toh-noh? |
| * intermittent? | * intermitente? | * een-**tehr**-mee-**tehn**-teh? |
| * mild? | * ligero? | * lee-**heh**-roh? |
| * moderate? | * moderado? | * moh-deh-**rah**-doh? |
| * severe? | * severo? | * seh-**veh**-roh? |
| * sharp? | * afilado? | * ah-fee-**lah**-doh? |
| * throbbing? | * pulsante? | * pool-**sahn**-teh |

| | | |
|---|---|---|
| *Do you feel like you have something in your eye?* | Siente como si tiene algo en su ojo? | **See-ehn**-teh **koh**-moh see **tee-eh**-neh **ahl**-goh ehn soo **oh**-hoh? |
| *Do you have headaches?* | Tiene dolores de cabeza? | **Tee-eh**-neh doh-**loh**-rehs deh kah-**beh**-sah? |
| *Do you have pain on movement of the eye?* | Tiene dolor al mover el ojo? | **Tee-eh**-neh doh-**lohr** ahl moh-**vehr** ehl **oh**-hoh? |
| *Does your brow hurt over that eye?* | Le duele la ceja sobre ese ojo? | Leh **dweh**-leh lah **seh**-hah **soh**-breh **eh**-seh **oh**-hoh? |
| *Have you had any injury to the eye?* | Se ha dañado el ojo? | Seh ah dah-**nyah**-doh ehl **oh**-hoh? |
| *Does anyone else in your family have a red eye?* | Hay alguién mas en su familia con el ojo rojo? | Ay ahl-**gee-ehn** mahs ehn soo fah-**mee**-lee-ah kohn ehl **oh**-hoh **roh**-hoh? |
| *Have you had any recent coughing spells?* | Ha tenido algún ataque de tos reciente? | Ah teh-**nee**-doh ahl-**goon** ah-**tah**-keh deh tohs reh-see-**ehn**-teh? |
| *Do you have a discharge from the eye?* | Tiene supuración del ojo? | **Tee-eh**-neh soo-poo-rah-**see-ohn** dehl **oh**-hoh? |
| *Do you get excessive tearing?* | Le llora excesivamente el ojo? | Leh **yoh**-rah eg-seh-**see**-vah-**mehn**-teh ehl **oh**-hoh? |

## Ears:

| English | Spanish | Pronunciation |
|---|---|---|
| Let me see in this ear. | Déjeme ver en éste oído. | **Deh**-heh-meh vehr ehn **ehs**-teh oh-**ee**-doh. |
| Let me see the other one. | Déjeme ver el otro. | **Deh**-heh-meh vehr ehl **oh**-troh. |
| Is the discharge: | Es la supuración: | Ehs lah soo-poo-rah-**see-ohn**: |
| * clear? | * clara? | * **klah**-rah? |
| * reddish? | * rojiza? | * roh-**hee**-sah? |
| * white? | * blanca? | * **blahn**-kah? |
| * yellow? | * amarilla? | * ah-mah-**ree**-yhah? |
| * thick? | * espeso? | * ehs-**peh**-soh? |
| * thin? | * denso/ralo? | * **dehn**-soh/**rah**-loh? |
| Have you had a discharge before? | Ha tenido supuración antes de hoy? | Ah teh-**nee**-doh soo-poo-rah-**see-ohn** **ahn**-tehs deh oy? |
| Have you recently had had a: | Ha tenido reciente-mente una: | Ah teh-**nee**-doh reh-**see-ehn**-teh-**mehn**-teh **oo**-nah: |
| * throat infection? | * infección de garganta? | * een-feg-**see-ohn** deh gahr-**gahn**-tah? |
| * ear infection? | * infección de oídos? | * een-feg-**see-ohn** deh oh-**ee**-dohs? |
| * head injury? | * daño en la cabeza? | * **dah**-nyoh ehn lah kah-**beh**-sah? |
| * ear injury? | * daño en el oído? | * **dah**-nyoh ehn ehl oh-**ee**-doh? |
| Have you been using any ear drops? | Ha usado gotas para el oído? | Ah oo-**sah**-doh **goh**-tahs **pah**-rah ehl oh-**ee**-doh? |
| Have you been swimming lately? | Ha estado nadando ultimamente? | Ah ehs-**tah**-doh nah-**dahn**-doh **ool**-tee-mah-**mehn**-teh? |
| Do you now have an earache? | Tiene ahora dolor de oído? | **Tee-eh**-neh ah-**oh**-rah doh-**lohr** deh oh-**ee**-doh? |
| Do you have a hearing loss? | Tiene sordera en el oído? | **Tee-eh**-neh sohr-**deh**-rah ehn ehl oh-**ee**-doh? |
| Is it only in one ear? | Es sólo en un oído? | Ehs **soh**-loh ehn oon oh-**ee**-doh? |

| English | Spanish | Pronunciation |
|---|---|---|
| *Did you notice a sudden loss?* | Notó la sordera de pronto? | Noh-**toh** lah sohr-**deh**-rah deh **prohn**-toh? |
| *Do you hear this tuning fork vibrating?* | Oye esto (diapasón) al vibrar? | **Oh**-yheh **ehs**-toh (dee-ah-pah-**sohn**) ahl vee-**brahr**? |
| *Which side do you hear best with?* | En que lado lo oye mejor? | Ehn keh **lah**-doh loh **oh**-yheh meh-**hohr**? |
| *Have you had a cold?* | Ha tenido un catarro? | Ah teh-**nee**-doh oon kah-**tah**-rhoh? |
| *Is there anyone in your family with a hearing loss?* | Hay alguien en su familia que esté sordo? | Ay ahl-**gee-ehn** ehn soo fah-**mee**-lee-ah keh ehs-**teh** **sohr**-doh? |
| *Are you taking any medications?* | Esta tomando alguna medicina? | Ehs-**tah** toh-**mahn**-doh ahl-**goo**-nah meh-dee-**see**-nah? |
| *Were you ever given the antibiotic called gentamicin or strep-tomycin?* | Le dieron algun dia el antibiótico llamado gentamicina o strep-tomicina? | Leh **dee-eh**-rohn ahl-**goon** dee-ah ehl ahn-tee-**bee-oh**-tee-koh yah-**mah**-doh **gehn**-tah-mee-**see**-nah oh ehs-trep-toh-mee-**see**-nah? |
| *Do you know if you are allergic to any medication?* | Sabe si es alérgico a alguna medicina? | **Sah**-beh see ehs ah-**lehr**-hee-koh ah ahl-**goo**-nah meh-dee-**see**-nah? |
| *Do you get:* | Le coge a usted: | Leh **koh**-heh ah oos-**tehd**: |
| * ringing in ears? | * zumbido en los oídos? | * soom-**bee**-doh ehn lohs oh-**ee**-dohs? |
| * crackling noises? | * ruidos en los oídos? | * **rwee**-dohs ehn lohs oh-**ee**-dohs? |
| * vertigo? | * vértigo? | * **vehr**-tee-goh? |
| *Have you had this sensation before?* | Ha tenido ésta sensacion antes? | Ah teh-**nee**-doh **ehs**-tah sehn-sah-**see-ohn** **ahn**-tehs? |
| *Have you had it for a long time?* | Lo ha tenido por mucho tiempo? | Loh ah teh-**nee**-doh pohr **moo**-choh **tee-ehm**-poh? |
| *Does it occur suddenly?* | Le ocurre de repente? | Leh oh-**koo**-rheh deh reh-**pehn**-teh? |
| *Do you get it when you are:* | Le ocurre cuando esta: | Leh oh-**koo**-rheh **kwahn**-doh ehs-**tah**: |
| * lying down? | * acostado? | * ah-kohs-**tah**-doh? |

| | | |
|---|---|---|
| * seating down? | * sentado? | * sehn-**tah**-doh? |
| * standing up? | * parado? | * pah-**rah**-doh? |
| *Does any position make you feel better/worse?* | Alguna posición lo hace sentir mejor/peor? | Ahl-**goo**-nah poh-see-**see-ohn** loh **ah**-seh sehn-**teer** meh-**hohr**/peh-**ohr**? |
| *During a vertigo attack have you noticed:* | Durante un ataque de vertigo ha notado: | Doo-**rahn**-teh oon ah-**tah**-keh deh **vehr**-tee-goh ah noh-**tah**-doh: |
| * a disturbance or gait? | * una molestia o paso poco seguro? | * **oo**-nah moh-**lehs**-tee-ah oh **pah**-soh **poh**-koh seh-**goo**-roh? |
| * decreased hearing? | * que oye menos? | * keh **oh**-yheh **meh**-nohs? |
| * double vision? | * visión doble? | * vee-**see-ohn doh**-bleh? |
| * loss of strength? | * perdida de fuerzas? | * **pehr**-dee-dah deh **fwehr**-sahs? |
| * nausea? | * nauseas? | * **nah**-oo-seh-ahs? |
| * ringing in your ears? | * zumbido en los oídos? | * soom-**bee**-doh ehn lohs oh-**ee**-dohs? |
| * vomiting? | * vomitos? | * **voh**-mee-tohs? |

Nose:

| | | |
|---|---|---|
| *Do you suffer from:* | Sufre usted de: | **Soo**-freh oos-**tehd** deh: |
| * allergies? | * alérgias? | * ah-**lehr**-hee-ahs? |
| * hay fever? | * alérgia al heno? | * ah-**lehr**-hee-ah ahl **eh**-noh? |
| *Is a postnasal drip present?* | Tiene presente un goteo nasal en la garganta? | **Tee-eh**-neh preh-**sehn**-teh oon goh-**teh-oh** nah-**sahl** ehn lah gahr-**gahn**-tah? |
| *Does your nose bleed easily?* | Le sangra su nariz con facilidad? | Leh **sahn**-grah soo nah-**reehs** kohn fah-see-lee-dad? |
| *Do you have a history of nasal polyps?* | Tiene historial de pólipos nasales? | **Tee-eh**-neh ees-toh-**ree-ahl** deh **poh**-lee-pohs nah-**sah**-lehs? |
| *How long have the polyps been present?* | Cuanto tiempo han estado los pólipos presente? | **Kwahn**-toh **tee-ehm**-poh ahn ehs-**tah**-doh lohs **poh**-lee- pohs preh-**sehn**-teh? |

| Is the obstruction affiliated with other symptoms? | Está la obstrucción asociada con otros síntomas? | Ehs-**tah** lah obs-troog-**see-ohn** ah-soh-**see-ah**-dah kohn **oh**-trohs **seen**-toh-mahs? |

Throat:

| Where exactly does your throat hurt? | Donde exáctamente le duele la garganta? | **Dohn**-deh eh-**sag**-tah-**mehn**-teh leh **dweh**-leh lah gahr-**gahn**-tah? |
| Is your throat: | Esta su garganta: | Ehs-**tah** soo gahr-**gahn**-tah: |
| * painful when you swallow? | * adolorida al tragar? | * ah-doh-loh-**ree**-dah ahl trah-**gahr**? |
| * scratchy? | * raspeante? | * **rahs**-peh-**ahn**-teh? |
| * with a dryness? | * con sequedad? | * kohn seh-**keh**-dad? |
| Do you frequently get: | Le da con frequencia: | Leh dah kohn freh-**kwehn**-see-ah: |
| * sore throats? | * dolor de garganta? | * doh-**lohr** deh gahr-**gahn**-tah? |
| * colds? | * resfriados? | * rehs-**free-ah**-dohs? |
| * strep throat? | * infección de garganta? | * een-feg-**see-ohn** deh gahr-**gahn**-tah? |
| I'm going to take a sample of your throat. | Voy a tomar una muestra de su garganta. | Voy ah toh-**mahr** **oo**-nah **mwehs**-trah deh soo gahr-**gahn**-tah. |
| Open your mouth wide and say aagghh. | Abra ancha su boca y diga aagghh. | **Ah**-brah **ahn**-chah soo **boh**-kah ee **dee**-gah aagghh. |
| You will feel a slight discomfort. | Va a sentir un poco de molestia. | Vah ah sehn-**teer** oon **poh**-koh deh moh-**lehs**-tee-ah. |
| You need to take some medicine. | Necesita tomar unas medicinas. | Neh-seh-**see**-tah toh-**mahr** **oo**-nahs meh-dee-**see**-nahs. |

Mouth:

| Open your mouth, please. | Abra la boca, por favor. | **Ah**-brah lah **boh**-kah, pohr fah-**vohr**. |
| Say aagghh! | Diga aahh! | **Dee**-gah aahh! |

| | | |
|---|---|---|
| *Swallow, please.* | Trage, por favor. | **Trah**-geh, pohr fah-**vohr**. |
| *Cough.* | Tosa. | **Toh**-sah. |
| *Do it again.* | Hágalo otra vez. | **Ah**-gah-loh **oh**-trah vehs. |
| *Stick out your tongue.* | Saque su lengua. | **Sah**-keh soo **lehn**-gwah. |
| *Do you have sores/ ulcers in your mouth?* | Tiene úlceras/llagas en su boca? | **Tee-eh**-neh **ool**-seh-rahs/ yah-**gahs** ehn soo **boh**-kah? |
| *Have you had them for long?* | Las ha tenido por mucho tiempo? | Lahs ah teh-**nee**-doh pohr moo-choh **tee-ehm**-poh? |
| *Do the lesions occur in groups?* | Ocurren las lesiones en grupos? | Oh-**koo**-rhehn lahs leh-**see-oh**-nehs ehn **groo**-pohs? |
| *Are the lesions painful?* | Son dolorosas las lesiones? | Sohn doh-loh-**roh**-sahs lahs leh-**see-oh**-nehs? |
| *Do you have bleeding gums?* | Tiene las encías sangrantes? | **Tee-eh**-neh lahs ehn-**see**-ahs sahn-**grahn**-tehs? |
| *Do you have sores in other parts of your body?* | Tiene llagas en otras partes del cuerpo? | **Tee-eh**-neh **yah**-gahs ehn **oh**-trahs **pahr**-tehs dehl **kwehr**-poh? |
| *Do you have them in the:* | Las tiene en el: | Lahs **tee-eh**-neh ehn ehl: |
| * anus? | * ano? | * **ah**-noh? |
| * urethra? | * uretra? | * oo-**reh**-trah? |
| * vagina? | * vagina? | * vah-**hee**-nah? |
| *Do you smoke?* | Fuma usted? | **Foo**-mah oos-**tehd**? |
| *If so... how much? (Please show me with your fingers.)* | Cuánto fuma? (Por favor, enséñeme con sus dedos.) | **Kwahn**-toh **foo**-mah? (Pohr fah-**vohr** ehn-**seh**-nyeh-meh kohn soos **deh**-dohs.) |
| *Are you taking any medications?* | Está tomando alguna medicina? | Ehs-**tah** toh-**mahn**-doh ahl **goo**-nah meh-dee-**see**-nah? |
| *Do you have a history of venereal disease?* | Tiene historial de enfermedades venéreas? | **Tee-eh**-neh ees-toh-**ree-ahl** deh **ehn**-fehr-meh-**dah**-dehs veh-**neh**-reh-ahs? |

Neck:

| | | |
|---|---|---|
| *Do you have or have* | Tiene ahora o ha | **Tee-eh**-neh ah-**oh**-rah oh |

33

| English | Spanish | Pronunciation |
|---|---|---|
| you ever had: | tenido antes: | ah teh-**nee**-doh **ahn**-tehs: |
| * enlarged glands? | * glándulas agrandadas? | * **glahn**-doo-lahs ah-grahn-**dah**-dahs? |
| * stiffness? | * rigidez? | * **ree**-hee-dehs? |
| * thyroid trouble? | * problemas del tiroide? | * proh-**bleh**-mahs dehl tee-**roy**-deh? |

## Larynx:

| English | Spanish | Pronunciation |
|---|---|---|
| *Have you ever had any injury to your neck?* | Ha sufrido alguna vez daño a su cuello? | Ah soo-**free**-doh ahl-**goo**-nah vehs **dah**-nyoh ah soo **kweh**-yoh? |
| *Have you noticed any swelling in your neck?* | Ha notado inflamación en su cuello? | Ah noh-**tah**-doh een-flah-mah-**see-ohn** ehn soo **kweh**-yoh? |
| *Do you suffer from frequent hoarseness?* | Sufre con frequencia de ronquera? | **Soo**-freh kohn freh-**kwehn**-see-ah deh rohn-**keh**-rah? |
| *Is there anything that makes it better?* | Hay algo que lo hace mejor? | Ay **ahl**-goh keh loh **ah**-seh meh-**hohr**? |
| *Is it worse/better in the daytime?* | Es peor/mejor durante el día? | Ehs peh-**ohr**/meh-**hohr** doo-**rahn**-teh ehl **dee**-ah? |

## Blood, Lymphatic:

| English | Spanish | Pronunciation |
|---|---|---|
| *Have you ever had:* | Ha tenido usted: | Ah teh-**nee**-doh oos-**tehd**: |
| * low blood count? | * conteo bajo de glóbulos rojos? | * kohn-**teh**-oh **bah**-hoh deh **gloh**-boo-lohs **roh**-hohs? |
| * anemia? | * anemia? | * ah-**neh**-mee-ah? |
| * blood transfusion? | * transfusión de sangre? | * trahns-foo-**see-ohn** deh **sahn**-greh? |
| *When you suffer a cut, do you bleed severely?* | Sangra en exceso cuando sufre una herida? | **Sahn**-grah ehn eg-**seh**-soh **kwahn**-doh soo-freh oo-nah eh-**ree**-dah? |
| *Have you felt any lumps in your:* | Ha sentido alguna masa en su: | Ah sehn-**tee**-doh ahl-**goo**-nah **mah**-sah ehn soo: |
| * groin? | * ingle? | * een-**gleh**? |
| * neck? | * cuello? | * **kweh**-yoh? |
| * armpit? | * axila/sobaco? | * ag-**see**-lah/soh-**bah**-koh? |
| * chest? | * pecho? | * **peh**-choh? |

| Are they (the lumps) painful? | Le duelen mucho las masas (protuberancias)? | Leh **dweh**-lehn **moo**-choh lahs **mah**-sahs (proh-too-beh-**rahn**-see-ahs)? |

## Chest:

| I will place this on your chest, it may be cold. (pointing to the stethoscope) | Voy a poner esto en su pecho, puede estar frio. | Voy ah poh-**nehr ehs**-toh ehn soo **peh**-choh, **pweh**-deh ehs-**tahr free**-oh. |
| I'm going to listen to your heart. | Voy a escuchar a su corazón. | Voy ah ehs-koo-**chahr** ah soo koh-rah-**sohn**. |
| Let me hear it on the back. | Déjeme escucharle atras. | **Deh**-heh-meh ehs-koo-**char**-leh ah-**trahs**. |
| Open your mouth and breathe in. | Abra su boca y respire profundo. | **Ah**-brah soo **boh**-kah ee rehs-**pee**-reh proh-**foon**-doh. |
| Open your mouth and breathe out. | Abra su boca y respire hacia afuera. | **Ah**-brah soo **boh**-kah ee rehs-**pee**-reh ah-see-ah ah-**fweh**-rah. |
| Relax. | Relajese. | Reh-**lah**-heh-seh. |
| Lie down. | Acuéstese. | Ah-**kwehs**-teh-seh. |
| Turn to the right. | Dése vuelta a la derecha. | **Deh**-seh **vwehl**-tah ah lah deh-**reh**-chah. |
| Turn to the left. | Dése vuelta a la izquierda. | **Deh**-seh **vwehl**-tah ah lah ees-**kee-ehr**-dah. |
| You may sit up. | Se puede sentar. | Seh **pweh**-deh sehn-**tahr**. |

## Cardiovascular:

| Have you experienced the palpitations for long time? | Hace mucho tiempo que le empezarón las palpitaciones? | **Ah**-seh **moo**-choh tee-**ehm**-poh keh leh ehm-peh-**sah**-rohn lahs pahl-pee-tah-**see-oh**-nehs? |
| Do they start suddenly? | Le empiezan de repente? | Leh ehm-**pee-eh**-sahn deh **reh-pehn**-teh? |
| Do they stop abruptly? | Se le terminan abruptamente? | Seh leh tehr-**mee**-nahn ah-**broop**-tah-**mehn**-teh? |
| Do they last a long time? | Le duran por mucho tiempo? | Leh **doo**-rahn pohr **moo**-choh **tee-ehm**-poh? |
| Can you do anything | Puede hacer algo que | **Pweh**-deh ah-**sehr ahl**-goh |

35

| | | |
|---|---|---|
| to stop the palpitations? | le pare las palpitaciones? | keh leh **pah**-reh lahs pahl-pee-tah-**see-oh**-nehs? |
| *Do you get these palpitations often?* | Le ocurren las palpitaciones con frequencia? | Leh oh-**koo**-rhen lahs pahl-pee-tah-**see-oh**-nehs kohn freh-**kwehn**-see-ah? |
| *How fast is your pulse during the attack?* | Durante el ataque, que de rapido es su pulso? | Doo-**rahn**-teh ehl ah-**tah**-keh, keh deh **rah**-pee-doh ehs soo **pool**-soh? |
| *Can you to tap out the rhythm on the table?* | Puede tocar el ritmo en la mesa? | **Pweh**-deh toh-**kahr** ehl **reet**-moh ehn lah **meh**-sah? |
| *Do you get the palpitations after:* | Le dan las palpitaciones despues de: | Leh dahn lahs pahl-pee-tah-**see-oh**-nehs dehs-**pwehs** deh: |
| * a meal? | * la comida? | * lah koh-**mee**-dah? |
| * exertion? | * hacer esfuerzo? | * ah-**sehr** ehs-**fwehr**-soh? |
| * strenuous exercise? | * hacer ejercicios vigoroso? | * ah-**sehr** eh-**hehr**-see-see-ohs vee-goh-**roh**-sohs? |
| * being tired? | * estar cansado? | * ehs-**tahr** kahn-**sah**-doh? |
| * while lying on your left side? | * cuando está acostado en su lado izquierdo? | * **kwahn**-doh ehs-**tah** ah-kohs-**tah**-doh ehn soo **lah**-doh ees-**kee-ehr**-doh? |
| *Have you fainted during the palpitations?* | Se ha desmayado durante las palpitaciones? | Seh ah dehs-mah-**yah**-doh doo-**rahn**-teh lahs pahl-pee-tah-**see-oh**-nehs? |
| *Do you have an intolerance to heat or cold?* | Tiene intolerancia al calor o frio? | **Tee-eh**-neh **een**-toh-leh-**rahn**-see-ah ahl kah-**lohr** oh free-oh? |
| *Do you take any medications?* | Toma alguna medicina? | **Toh**-mah ahl-**goo**-nah meh-dee-**see**-nah? |
| *Do you suffer from shortness of breath?* | Sufre de falta de aliento? | **Soo**-freh deh **fahl**-tah deh ah-**lee-ehn**-toh? |
| *Do you sleep on one pillow? Two?* | Duerme con una almohada? Dos? | **Dwehr**-meh kohn **oo**-nah ahl-**moh-ah**-dah? Dohs? |
| *Do you awaken at night short of breath?* | Se despierta en la noche con falta de aliento? | Seh dehs-**pee-ehr**-tah ehn lah **noh**-cheh kohn **fahl**-tah deh ah-**lee-ehn**-toh? |
| *Do you get chest pain?* | Le coge dolor en el | Leh **koh**-heh doh-**lohr** ehn |

| | | |
|---|---|---|
| Do you get the pain frequently? | Le coge el dolor con frequencia? | Leh **koh**-heh ehl doh-**lohr** kohn freh-**kwehn**-see-ah? |
| Does the pain last for a long time? | Le dura el dolor por mucho tiempo? | Leh **doo**-rah ehl doh-**lohr** pohr **moo**-choh tee-**ehm**-poh? |
| Does any of the following make it better: | Alguno de los siguientes lo hace sentir mejor: | Ahl-**goo**-noh deh lohs see-**gee-ehn**-tehs loh **ah**-seh sehn-**teer** meh-**hohr**: |
| * breathing? | * el respirar? | * ehl rehs-pee-**rahr**? |
| * lying flat? | * el acostarse? | * ehl ah-kohs-**tahr**-seh? |
| * moving your arms or neck? | * el mover su cuello o nuca? | * ehl moh-**vehr** soo **kweh**-yoh oh **noo**-kah? |
| * sitting up? | * el sentarse? | * ehl sehn-**tahr**-seh? |
| Would you say the pain is: | Diria usted que el dolor es: | Dee-**ree-ah** oos-**tehd** keh ehl doh-**lohr** ehs: |
| * aching? | * doloroso? | * doh-loh-**roh**-soh? |
| * burning? | * ardiente? | * ahr-**dee-ehn**-teh? |
| * constricting? | * estrujante? | * ehs-troo-**hahn**-teh? |
| * crushing? | * aplastante? | * ah-plahs-**tahn**-teh? |
| * dull? | * monótono? | * moh-**noh**-toh-noh? |
| * pressing? | * apretante? | * ah-preh-**tahn**-teh? |
| * sharp? | * afilado? | * ah-fee-**lah**-doh? |
| * throbbing? | * pulsante? | * pool-**sahn**-teh? |
| Does the pain develop: | Empieza el dolor: | Ehm-**pee-eh**-sah ehl doh-**lohr**: |
| * after eating? | * despues de comer? | * dehs-**pwehs** deh koh-**mehr**? |
| * during sexual intercourse? | * cuando hace el amor? | * **kwahn**-doh **ah**-seh ehl ah-**mohr**? |
| * at rest? | * cuando descansa? | * **kwahn**-doh dehs-**kahn**-sah? |
| * when moving your arms? | * cuando mueve sus brazos? | * **kwahn**-doh **mweh**-veh soos **brah**-sohs? |

| | | |
|---|---|---|
| * when sleeping? | * cuando duerme? | * **kwahn**-doh **dwehr**-meh? |
| * with emotional strain? | * con tensión emocional? | * kohn tehn-**see-ohn** eh-moh-**see-oh**-nahl? |
| * with exertion? | * con esfuerzo? | * kohn ehs-**fwher**-soh? |
| *Is the pain associated with:* | Esta el dolor asociado con: | Ehs-**tah** ehl doh-**lohr** ah-soh-**see-ah**-doh kohn: |
| * coughing up blood? | * el tocer sangre? | * ehl toh-**sehr sahn**-greh? |
| * coughing? | * tocer? | * toh-**sehr**? |
| * fever? | * fiebre? | * **fee-eh**-breh? |
| * leg pain? | * dolor en la pierna? | * doh-**lohr** ehn lah **pee-ehr**-nah? |
| * nausea? | * nauseas? | * **nah**-oo-seh-ahs? |
| * palpitations? | * palpitaciones? | * **pahl**-pee-tah-see-**oh**-nehs? |
| * shortness of breath? | * falta de aliento? | * **fahl**-tah deh ah-**lee-ehn**-toh? |
| * vomiting? | * vomitos? | * **voh**-mee-tohs? |
| *Have you noticed a blue color (cyanosis) on your:* | Ha notado algún color color azul en sus: | Ah noh-**tah**-doh ahl-**goon** koh-**lohr** ah-**sool** ehn soos: |
| * lips? | * labios? | * **lah**-bee-ohs? |
| * nails? | * uñas? | * **oo**-nyahs? |
| * skin? | * piel? | * pee-ehl? |
| * anywhere else? | * en otro lugar? | * ehn **oh**-troh loo-**gahr**? |
| *Please show me where.* | Por favor enséñeme donde? | Pohr fah-**vohr** ehn-**seh**-nyeh-meh **dohn**-deh? |
| *Do you know of any _____ problem?* | Sabe de algun problema _____ | **Sah**-beh deh ahl-**goon** proh-**bleh**-mah _____ |
| * blood | * de la sangre? | * deh la **sahn**-greh? |
| * heart | * del corazón? | * dehl koh-rah-**sohn**? |
| * lung | * de los pulmones? | * deh lohs pool-**moh**-nehs? |
| *How long has the* | Por cuanto tiempo ha | Pohr **kwahn**-toh **tee-ehm**- |

| | | |
|---|---|---|
| blue color (cyanosis) been present? | tenido el color azúl (la cianosis)? | poh ah teh-**nee**-doh ehl koh-**lohr** ah-**sool** (lah see-ah-**noh**-sees)? |
| *Does anything make the color better?* | Hay algo que mejore el color? | Ay **ahl**-goh keh meh-**hoh**-reh ehl koh-**lohr**? |
| *Does anything make the color worse?* | Hay algo que empeóre el color? | Ay **ahl**-goh keh ehm-peh-**oh**-reh ehl koh-**lohr**? |
| *Is the cyanosis associated with:* | El color azúl está asociado con: | Ehl koh-**lohr** ah-**sool** ehs-**tah** ah-soh-**see-ah**-doh kohn: |
| * bleeding? | * el sangrar? | * ehl sahn-**grahr**? |
| * coughing? | * el tocer? | * ehl toh-**sehr**? |
| * shortness of breath? | * la falta de aliento? | * lah **fahl**-tah deh ah-**lee-ehn**-toh? |
| *Do you have a history of heart murmur?* | Tiene historial de murmullos del corazón? | **Tee-eh**-neh ees-**toh**-ree-ahl deh moor-**moo**-yohs dehl koh-rah-**sohn**? |
| *Do you suffer from hypertension?* | Sufre de hipertensión? | **Soo**-freh deh ee-pehr-tehn-**see-ohn**? |
| *Does anyone else in your family become cyanotic?* | Hay alguien en su familia que sea cianótico? | Ay **ahl**-gee-ehn ehn soo fah-**mee**-lee-ah keh **seh**-ah see-ah-**noh**-tee-koh? |
| *What type of work do you do?* | Que clase de trabajo hace? | Keh **klah**-seh deh trah-**bah**-hoh **ah**-seh? |
| *Do your feet/ankles get swollen?* | Se le inflaman sus pies/tobillos? | Seh leh een-**flah**-mahn soos pee-ehs/toh-**bee**-yohs? |
| *Have you had the swelling for long?* | Ha tenido la inflamación por mucho tiempo? | Ah teh-**nee**-doh lah een-flah-mah-**see-ohn** pohr **moo**-choh **tee-ehm**-poh? |
| *Did the swelling appear:* | La inflamación apareció de: | Lah **een**-flah-mah-**see-ohn** ah-pah-reh-**see-oh** deh: |
| * suddenly? | * pronto? | * **prohn**-toh? |
| * gradually? | * gradualmente? | * grah-dwahl-**mehn**-teh? |
| *Is the swelling worse as the day progresses?* | La inflamación se empeora mientras avanza el dia? | Lah **eeh**-flah-mah-**see-ohn** seh ehm-peh-**oh**-rah **mee-ehn**-trahs ah-**vahn**-sah ehl **dee**-ah? |

| | | |
|---|---|---|
| Does it disappear after a good night's rest? | Desaparece despues de dormir bien la noche? | **Deh**-sah-pah-**reh**-seh dehs-**pwehs** deh dohr-**meer** bee-ehn lah **noh**-cheh? |
| Does it disappear upon elevating your feet? | Desaparece cuando eleva sus pies? | Deh-sah-pah-**reh**-seh **kwahn**-doh eh-**leh**-vah soos pee-ehs? |
| Have you had the following diseases: | Ha tenido enferme-dades del: | Ah teh-**nee**-doh ehn-**fehr**-meh-**dah**-dehs dehl: |
| * kidney? | * riñón? | * ree-**nyohn**? |
| * heart? | * corazón? | * koh-rah-**sohn**? |
| * liver? | * hígado? | * **ee**gah-doh? |
| Do you suffer from pain in your legs? | Sufre de dolor en sus piernas? | Soo-freh deh doh-**lohr** ehn soos **pee-ehr**-nahs? |
| Have you noticed any ulcers on your legs? | Ha notado llagas en sus piernas? | Ah noh-**tah**-doh **yah**-gahs ehn soos **pee-ehr**-nahs? |
| Are you taking any oral contraceptives? | Está tomando algún anticonceptivo? | Ehs-**tah** toh-**mahn**-doh ahl-**goon ahn**-tee-kohn-**sep-tee**-voh? |
| Is the swelling asso-ciated with menstrual changes? | Ha notado hinchazón durante su menstrua-ción? | Ah noh-**tah**-doh een-chah-**sohn** doo-**rahn**-teh soo mehns-troo-ah-**see-ohn**? |

Pulmonary:

| | | |
|---|---|---|
| Does the shortness of breath appear suddenly or gradually? | La falta de aliento le empieza de pronto o gradualmente? | Lah **fahl**-tah deh ah-lee-**ehn**-toh leh ehm-**pee-eh**-sah deh **prohn**-toh oh grah-dwahl-**mehn**-teh? |
| Is it a constant shortness of breath? | Es constante la falta de aliento? | Ehs kohns-**tahn**-teh lah **fahl**-tah deh ah-lee-**ehn**-toh? |
| Does the shortness of breath occur: | La falta de aliento le ocurre cuando: | Lah **fahl**-tah deh ah-lee-**ehn**-toh leh oh-**koo**-rheh **kwahn**-doh: |
| * at rest? | * descansa? | * dehs-**kahn**-sah? |
| * lying flat? | * se acuesta? | * seh ah-**kwehs**-tah? |
| * sitting up? | * está sentado? | * ehs-**tah** sehn-**tah**-doh? |
| * with exertion? | * hace esfuerzo? | * **ah**-seh ehs-**fwher**-soh? |
| How many level blocks | Cuantas cuadras puede | **Kwahn**-tahs **kwah**-drahs |

40

| English | Spanish | Pronunciation |
|---|---|---|
| can you walk? | caminar? | **pweh**-deh kah-**mee**-nahr? |
| *Is the shortness of breath accompanied by any of the following:* | Le coge la falta de aliento con uno de los siguientes: | Leh **koh**-heh lah **fahl**-tah deh ah-lee-**ehn**-toh kohn **oo**-noh deh lohs see-**gee-ehn**-tehs: |
| * coughing up blood? | * tociendo sangre? | * toh-**see-ehn**-doh **sahn**-greh? |
| * cough? | * tos? | * tohs? |
| * hoarseness? | * ronquéra? | * rohn-**keh**-rah? |
| * palpitations? | * palpitaciones? | * **pahl**-pee-tah-**see-oh**-nehs? |
| * wheezing? | * sonido asmático? | * soh-**nee**-doh ahs-**mah**-tee-koh? |
| *How old were you when the wheezing started?* | Que edad tenia cuando le empezó el sonido asmático? | Keh eh-**dah** teh-**nee-ah kwahn**-doh leh ehm-peh-**soh** ehl soh-**nee**-doh ahs-**mah**-tee-koh? |
| *How frequently does the wheezing occur?* | Con que frequencia le ocurre el sonido? | Kohn keh freh-**kwehn**-see-ah leh oh-**koo**-rheh ehl soh-**nee**-doh? |
| *Is the wheezing caused by any of the following:* | Es causado el sonido por uno de los siquientes: | Ehs kah-oo-**sah**-do ehl soh-**nee**-doh pohr **oo**-noh deh lohs see-**gee-ehn**-tehs: |
| * animals? | * animales? | * ah-nee-**mah**-lehs? |
| * emotions? | * emociones? | * eh-moh-**see-oh**-nehs? |
| * food? | * comida? | * koh-**mee**-dah? |
| * odors? | * olores? | * oh-**loh**-rehs? |
| * weather? | * la temperatura? | * lah tehm-peh-rah-**too**-rah? |
| *Do you take any medication for it?* | Toma alguna medicina para ello? | **Toh**-mah ahl-**goo**-nah meh-dee-**see**-nah **pah**-rah **eh**-yhoh? |
| *Have the symptoms gotten better or worse over the years?* | Con los años se han mejorado o empeorado los síntomas? | Kohn lohs **ah**-nyohs seh ahn **meh**-hoh-**rah**-doh oh **ehm**-peh-oh-**rah**-doh lohs **seen**-toh-mahs? |
| *Have you had this* | Ha tenido esta tos por | Ah teh-**nee**-doh **ehs**-tah |

| cough for a long time? | mucho tiempo? | tohs pohr **moo**-choh **tee-ehm**-poh? |
|---|---|---|
| *Did you suddenly start coughing?* | Empezó a tocer de pronto? | Ehm-peh-**soh** ah toh-**sehr** deh **prohn**-toh? |
| *Are you a smoker?* | Fuma usted? | **Foo**-mah oos-**tehd**? |
| *How much do you smoke* | Cuánto fuma? | **Kwahn**-toh **foo**-mah? |
| *Do you produce phlegm when coughing?* | Produce flema cuando toce? | Proh-**doo**-seh **fleh**-mah **kwahn**-doh **toh**-seh? |
| *Is the color:* | Es el color: | Ehs ehl koh-**lohr**: |
| * clear? | * claro? | * **klah**-roh? |
| * yellow? | * amarillo? | * **ah**-mah-**ree**-yhoh? |
| * white? | * blanco? | * **blahn**-koh? |
| *Does it have a foul odor?* | Tiene mal olor la flema? | **Tee-eh**-neh mahl oh-**lohr** lah **fleh**-mah? |
| *Does the cough or coughing up of blood occur:* | La tos o el tocer sangre le ocurre: | Lah tohs oh ehl toh-**sehr** **sahn**-greh leh oh-**koo**-rheh: |
| * after eating? | * despues de comer? | * dehs-**pwehs** deh koh-**mehr**? |
| * while seating down? | * mientras está sentado? | * **mee-ehn**-trahs ehs-**tah** sehn-**tah**-doh? |
| * when sleeping? | * cuando duerme? | * **kwahn**-doh **dwehr**-meh? |
| * when exerting? | * cuando hace esfuerzo? | * **kwahn**-doh **ah**-seh ehs-**fwehr**-soh? |
| * in any position? | * en cualquier posición? | * ehn kwahl-kee-ehr poh-see-**see-ohn**? |
| *Is there anything that relieves the cough?* | Hay algo que le alivia la tos? | Ay **ahl**-goh keh leh ah-**lee**-vee-ah lah tohs? |
| *Do you have other symptoms like:* | Tiene otros síntomas como: | **Tee-eh**-neh **oh**-trohs **seen**-toh-mahs **koh**-moh: |
| * back pains? | * dolor de espalda? | * doh-**lohr** deh ehs-**pal**-dah? |
| * chest pains? | * dolor del pecho? | * doh-**lohr** dehl **peh**-choh? |
| * fever? | * fiebre? | * **fee-eh**-breh? |

| | | |
|---|---|---|
| * headaches? | * dolor de cabeza? | * doh-**lohr** deh kah-**beh**-sah? |
| * hoarseness? | * ronquera? | * rohn-**keh**-rah? |
| * loss of consciousness? | * pérdida del conocimiento? | * **pehr**-dee-dah dehl koh-noh-see-**mee**-ehn-toh? |
| * runny nose? | * moqueadera? | * **moh**-keh-ah-**deh**-rah? |
| * shortness of breath? | * falta de aliento? | * **fahl**-tah deh ah-lee-**ehn**-toh? |
| * weight loss? | * pérdida de peso? | * **pehr**-dee-dah deh **peh**-soh? |
| *Do you have pets?* | Tiene animales? | **Tee-eh**-neh ah-nee-**mah**-lehs? |
| *Do you know if you have been exposed to tuberculosis?* | Sabe si ha sido expuesto a la tuberculosis? | **Sah**-beh see ah **see**-doh egs-**pwehs**-toh ah lah too-behr-koo-**loh**-sees? |
| *Have you noticed any blood in your phlegm (sputum)?* | Ha notado alguna sangre en su flema? | Ah noh-**tah**-doh ahl-**goo**-nah **sahn**-greh ehn soo **fleh**-mah? |
| *Do you actually see clots of blood in your sputum?* | Ve usted coágulos de sangre en su esputo? | Veh oos-**tehd** koh-**ah**-goo-lohs deh **sahn**-greh ehn soo ehs-**poo**-toh? |
| *Have you been coughing up blood for a long time?* | Ha estado tociendo sangre por mucho tiempo? | Ah ehs-**tah**-doh toh-**see**-**ehn**-doh **sahn**-greh pohr **moo**-choh **tee-ehm**-poh? |
| *Are you taking any blood thinners?* | Está tomando algo para disminuir la sangre? | Ehs-**tah** toh-**mahn**-doh **ahl**-goh **pah**-rah **dees**-mee-noo-eer lah **sahn**-greh? |
| *Is there a history of heart disease?* | Padece del corazón? | Pah-**deh**-seh dehl koh-rah-**sohn**? |

Breasts:

| | | |
|---|---|---|
| *Do you know how to examine your breasts?* | Sabe como examinarse los senos? | **Sah**-beh **koh**-moh eg-sah-mee-**nahr**-seh lohs **seh**-nohs? |
| *Do you examine your breasts every month?* | Se examina el seno cada mes? | Seh eg-sah-**mee**-nah ehl **seh**-noh **kah**-dah mehs? |
| *Show me how you do it.* | Enséñeme como lo hace. | Ehn-**seh**-nyeh-meh **koh**-moh loh **ah**-seh. |
| *Have you ever noticed* | Ha notado antes una | Ah noh-**tah**-doh **ahn**-tehs |

| English | Spanish | Pronunciation |
|---|---|---|
| a mass (lump) before? | masa (protuberancia)? | **oo**-nah **mah**-sah (proh-too-beh-**rahn**-see-ah)? |
| *Does it change in size* during your menstrual cycle? | Cambia la masa de tamaño durante la menstruación? | **Kahm**-bee-ah lah **mah**-sah deh tah-**mah**-nyoh doo-**rahn**-teh lah **mens**-troo-ah-**see-ohn**? |
| *I need to examine* your breasts. | Necesito examinarle los senos. | Neh-seh-**see**-toh eg-sah-mee-**nahr**-leh lohs **seh**-nohs. |
| *Has there been a* change of skin color on the breast? | Ha habido cambio en el color del seno? | Ah ah-**bee**-doh **kahm**-bee-oh ehn ehl koh-**lohr** dehl **seh**-noh? |
| *Have you ever suffered* a breast injury? | Ha sufrido algún daño al seno? | Ah soo-**free**-doh **ahl**-goon **dah**-nyoh ahl **seh**-noh? |
| *Are your breasts or* nipples: | Están sus senos o pezones: | Ehs-**tahn** soos **seh**-nohs oh peh-**soh**-nehs: |
| * tender? | * lastimosos? | * lahs-tee-**moh**-sohs? |
| * painful? | * adoloridos? | * ah-doh-loh-**ree**-dohs? |
| * discharging? | * supurando? | * soo-poo-**rahn**-doh? |
| *Does the pain in your* breasts get better/worse with your menstrual cycle? | Se mejora/empeora el dolor en los senos con su menstruación? | Seh meh-**hoh**-rah/ehm-peh-**oh**-rah ehl doh-**lohr** ehn lohs **seh**-nohs kon soo **mens**-troo-ah-**see-ohn**? |
| *What is the color of* the discharge? | De que color es la supuración? | Deh keh koh-**lohr** ehs lah soo-poo-rah-**see-ohn**? |
| *Do you get a discharge* from both breasts? | Le supuran ambos senos? | Leh soo-**poo**-rahn **ahm**-bohs **seh**-nohs? |
| *Do you only get the* discharge during your menstrual cycle? | Tiene la supuración sólo durante la menstruación? | **Tee-eh**-neh lah soo-poo-rah-**see-ohn** soh-loh doo-**rahn**-teh lah **mens**-troo-ah-**see-ohn**? |
| *Is the discharge associated with breast tenderness?* | Le coge la supuración cuando el seno esta lastimoso? | Le **koh**-heh lah **soo**-poo-rah-**see-ohn kwahn**-doh ehl **seh**-noh ehs-**tah** lahs-tee-**moh**-soh? |
| *Are you taking any* oral contraceptives? | Está tomando algún anticonceptivo? | Ehs-**tah** toh-**mahn**-doh ahl-**goon** ahn-tee-kohn-**sep**-tee-voh? |
| *Did you have any* problems with your | Tuvo algún problema con su último embarazo | **Too**-voh ahl-**goon** proh-**bleh**-mah kohn soo **ool-** |

| | | |
|---|---|---|
| last pregnancy and delivery? | y parto? | tee-moh-ehm-bah-**rah**-soh ee **pahr**-toh? |
| *Has your brassiere size changed any?* | Ha cambiado la talla de su sugetador (brasier)? | Ah kahm-**bee-ah**-doh lah **tah**-yah deh soo soo-heh-tah-dohr (brah-see-ehr)? |

Abdomen:

| | | |
|---|---|---|
| *Do you get abdominal pain?* | Le dan dolores en el abdomen? | Leh dahn doh-**loh**-rehs ehn ehl ab-doh-**mehn**? |
| *Show me where the pain is located.* | Enséñeme donde esta localizado el dolor. | Ehn-**seh**-nyeh-meh **dohn**-deh ehs-**tah** loh-kah-lee-**sah**-doh ehl doh-**lohr**. |
| *Has it changed location since it started?* | Ha cambiado de lugar el dolor desde que empezo? | Ah kahm-**bee-ah**-doh deh loo-**gahr** ehl doh-**lohr** **dehs**-deh keh ehm-peh-**soh**? |
| *Is the pain associated with:* | Está el dolor asociado con: | Ehs-**tah** ehl doh-**lohr** ah-soh-**see-ah**-doh kohn: |
| * abdominal distention? | * inflamación abdominal? | * een-flah-mah-**see-ohn** ab-doh-mee-**nahl**? |
| * bloody stools? | * excrementos sanguíneos? | * egs-kreh-**mehn**-tohs sahn-**gee**-neh-ohs? |
| * chills? | * escalofrios? | * ehs-kah-loh-**free-ohs**? |
| * constipation? | * estreñimiento? | * **ehs**-treh-nyee-**mee-ehn**-toh? |
| * diarrhea? | * diarrea? | * dee-ah-**rheh-ah**? |
| * eating? | * el comer? | * ehl koh-**mehr**? |
| * fever? | * fiebre? | * **fee-eh**-breh? |
| * nausea? | * nausea? | * **nah**-oo-seh-ah? |
| * sweating? | * sudor? | * soo-**dohr**? |
| * vomiting? | * vomitos? | * **voh**-mee-tohs? |
| *Is the pain:* | Es el dolor: | Ehs ehl doh-**lohr**: |
| * burning? | * ardiente? | * ahr-**dee-ehn**-teh? |
| * continuous? | * continuo? | * konh-**tee**-noo-oh? |
| * cramping? | * retortijante? | * reh-tohr-**tee**-hahn-teh? |

| | | |
|---|---|---|
| * sharp? | * afilado? | * ah-fee-**lah**-doh? |
| *Please lie down here.* | Por favor acuéstese aqui. | Pohr fah-**vohr** ah-**kwehs**-teh-seh ah-**kee**. |
| *Relax your stomach muscles.* | Relaje su estómago. | Reh-**lah**-heh soo ehs-**toh**-mah-goh. |
| *Tell me if you feel any pain when I press.* | Digame si siente algún dolor cuando empujo. | Dee-gah-meh see **see-ehn**-teh ahl-**goon** doh-**lohr** **kwahn**-doh ehm-**poo**-hoh. |
| *Does it hurt here?* | Le duele aqui? | Leh **dweh**-leh ah-**kee**? |
| *Does it hurt when I let go?* | Le duele cuando le suelto? | Leh **dweh**-leh **kwahn**-doh leh **swehl**-toh? |
| *Turn to the right.* | Dése vuelta a la derecha. | **Deh**-seh vwehl-tah ah lah deh-**reh**-chah. |
| *Turn to the left.* | Dése vuelta a la izquierda. | **Deh**-seh vwehl-tah ah lah ees-**kee-ehr**-dah. |
| *Please relax; calm down.* | Por favor, relájese; calmese. | Pohr fah-**vohr**, reh-**lah**-heh-seh; **kahl**-meh-seh. |
| *Please, stand up.* | Por favor, párece. | Pohr fah-**vohr**, **pah**-reh-seh. |
| *Sit down/Sit up.* | Siéntese. | **See-ehn**-teh-seh. |
| *Do you have difficulty swallowing?* | Tiene dificultad al tragar? | **Tee-eh**-neh dee-fee-kool-tad ahl trah-**gahr**? |
| *Has your appetite changed?* | Le ha cambiado su apetito? | Leh ah kahm-**bee-ah**-doh soo ah-peh-**tee**-toh? |
| *Do you often have indigestion?* | Le da mala digestión con frequencia? | Leh dah **mah**-lah dee-hehs-**tee-ohn** kohn freh-**kwehn**-see-ah? |
| *Do you burp a lot?* | Eructa mucho? | Eh-**roog**-tah **moo**-choh? |
| *Do you get gas pain?* | Suele tener dolor de gas? | **Sweh**-leh teh-**nehr** doh-**lohr** de gahs? |
| *Do you get heartburn?* | Le coge acedia (acedez)? | Leh **koh**-heh ah-seh-**dee**-ah (ah-seh-**dehs**)? |
| *Do you get frequent stomach aches?* | Tiene con frequencia dolor estomacal? | **Tee-eh**-neh kohn freh-**kwehn**-see-ah doh-**lohr** ehs-toh-mah-**kahl**? |
| *Have you ever had an ulcer?* | Alguna vez ha tenido úlcera? | Ahl-**goo**-nah vehs ah teh-**nee**-doh **ool**-seh-rah? |

| Do you take medicine for your stomach? | Toma medicina para el estómago? | **Toh**-mah meh-dee-**see**-nah **pah**-rah ehl ehs-**toh**-mah-goh? |
|---|---|---|
| Do you have the bottle with you? | Tiene la botella con usted? | **Tee-eh**-neh lah boh-**teh**-yhah kohn oos-**tehd**? |
| Please show me the bottle. | Por favor enséñeme la botella. | Pohr fah-**vohr** ehn-**seh**-nyeh-meh lah boh-**teh**-yhah. |
| Do you remember the name? | Se acuerda del nombre? | Seh ah-**kwehr**-dah dehl **nohm**-breh? |
| Please write it down here. | Por favor escríbalo aquí. | Pohr fah-**vohr** ehs-**kree**-bah-loh ah-**kee**. |
| Have you gained any weight lately? | Ha subido de peso últimamente? | Ah soo-**bee**-doh deh **peh**-soh **ool**-tee-mah-**mehn**-teh? |
| Has there been a change in your bowel habits recently? | Ha habido un cambio reciente en su defecación habitual? | Ah ah-**bee**-doh oon **kahm**-bee-oh reh-**see-ehn**-teh ehn soo deh-feh-kah-**see-ohn** ah-bee-**twahl**? |
| Are you constipated? | Está usted estreñido? | Ehs-**tah** oos-**tehd** ehs-treh-**nyee**-doh? |
| When was your last bowel movement? | Cuando fué su última evacuación de excremento? | **Kwahn**-doh **fweh** soo **ool**-tee-mah eh-vah-kwah-**see-ohn** deh egs-kreh-**mehn**-toh? |
| Did you take a laxative? | Tomó un purgante/laxante? | Toh-**moh** oon poor-**gahn**-teh/lag-**sahn**-teh? |
| Did the jaundice occur gradually or suddenly? | La ictericia amarilla le ocurrió de repente o gradual? | Lah eeg-teh-**ree**-see-ah ah-mah-**ree**-yhah leh oh-koo-**ree-oh** deh reh-**pehn**-teh oh grah-dwahl? |
| Is it associated with: | Esta asociada con: | Ehs-**tah** ah-soh-**see-ah**-dah kohn: |
| * abdominal pain? | * dolor abdominal? | * doh-**lohr** ab-doh-mee-nahl? |
| * anal discomfort? | * molestia anal? | * moh-**lehs**-tee-ah ah-**nahl**? |
| * belching? | * eructos? | * eh-roog-tohs? |
| * black tarry stool? | * excremento color alquitrán negro? | * egs-kreh-**mehn**-toh koh-**lohr**-ahl-kee-**trahn** neh-groh? |

47

| | | |
|---|---|---|
| * bloating? | * hinchazón? | * een-chah-**sohn**? |
| * change in abdominal girth? | * cambio en su cintura? | * **kahm**-bee-oh ehn soo seen-**too**-rah? |
| * change in bowel habits? | * cambio en su defecación habitual? | * **kahm**-bee-oh ehn soo **deh**-feh-kah-**see-ohn** ah-bee-too-ahl? |
| * constipation? | * estreñimiento? | * **ehs**-treh-nyee-**mee-ehn**-toh? |
| * diarrhea? | * diarrea? | * dee-ah-**rheh-ah**? |
| * hemorrhoids? | * hemorroides? | * eh-moh-roy-dehs? |
| * hepatitis? | * hepatitis? | * eh-pah-**tee**-tees? |
| * hernia? | * hernia? | * **ehr**-nee-ah? |
| * loss of appetite? | * perdida de apetito? | * **perh**-dee-dah deh ah-peh-**tee**-toh? |
| * nausea? | * nauseas? | * **nah**-oo-seh-ahs? |
| * parasites? | * parásitos? | * pah-**rah**-see-tohs? |
| * change in stool shape and color? | * cambio de color y forma del excremento? | * **kahm**-bee-oh deh koh-**lohr** ee **fohr**-mah dehl egs-kreh-**mehn**-toh? |
| * vomiting blood? | * vomitos de sangre? | * **voh**-mee-tohs deh **sahn**-greh? |
| * vomiting? | * vomitos? | * **voh**-mee-tohs? |

Genital and Urinary:

| | | |
|---|---|---|
| *Do you urinate often?* | Orina con frequencia? | Oh-**ree**-nah kohn freh-**kwehn**-see-ah? |
| *How many times a day* do you urinate? | Cuántas veces al dia orina usted? | **Kwahn**-tahs **veh**-sehs ahl **dee**-ah oh-**ree**-nah oos-**tehd**? |
| *Do you have pain* or burning with urination? | Tiene usted dolor o ardor cuando orina? | **Tee-eh**-neh oos-**tehd** doh-**lohr** oh ahr-**dohr kwahn**-doh oh-**ree**-nah? |
| *Does the pain radiate* toward: | Se corre el dolor hacia: | Seh **koh**-rheh ehl doh-**lohr** ah-see-ah: |
| * the back? | * la espalda? | * lah ehs-**pahl**-dah? |

| English | Spanish | Pronunciation |
|---|---|---|
| * the groin? | * el ingle? | * ehl **een**-gleh? |
| *Do you drink lots of liquid?* | Tóma mucho líquido? | **Toh**-mah **moo**-choh **lee**-kee-doh? |
| *During the night do you get up to urinate?* | Se levanta en la noche a orinar? | Seh leh-**vahn**-tah ehn lah **noh**-cheh ah oh-**ree**-nahr? |
| *Show me with your finger how many times.* | Enséñeme con sus dedos cuantas veces. | Ehn-**seh**-nyeh-meh kohn soos **deh**-dohs **kwahn**-tahs **veh**-sehs. |
| *Is the flow strong and continuous?* | Es fuerte y contínuo el chorro de orina? | Ehs **fwehr**-teh ee kohn-**tee**-noo-oh ehl **choh**-rroh deh oh-**ree**-nah? |
| *Is there any change to the flow from day to night?* | Hay algún cambio en el chorro del día a la noche? | Ay ahl-**goon kahm**-bee-oh ehn ehl **choh**-rroh dehl **dee**-ah ah lah **noh**-cheh? |
| *Have you noticed blood in your urine?* | Ha notado sangre en su orina? | Ah noh-**tah**-doh **sahn**-greh ehn soo oh-**ree**-nah? |
| *Has it been:* | Ha sido: | Ah **see**-doh: |
| * just a few drops? | * unas pocas gotas? | * **oo**-nahs **poh**-kahs **goh**-tahs? |
| * pure blood? | * pura sangre? | * **poo**-rah **sahn**-greh? |
| *Is the urine:* | Es la orina: | Ehs lah oh-**ree**-nah: |
| * bloody? | * sangrienta? | * sahn-**gree-ehn**-tah? |
| * clear? | * clara? | * **klah**-rah? |
| * cloudy? | * turbia? | * **toor**-bee-ah? |
| * dark? | * oscura? | * ohs-**koo**-rah? |
| * odorous? | * mal oliente? | * mahl oh-**lee-ehn**-teh? |
| *Do you ever lose urine when:* | Pierde usted orina cuando: | **Pee-ehr**-deh oos-**tehd** oh-**ree**-nah **kwahn**-doh: |
| * coughing? | * toce? | * toh-seh? |
| * laughing? | * se ríe? | * seh **ree**-eh? |
| * exercising? | * hace ejercicios? | * **ah**-seh eh-**hehr**-see-**see-ohs**? |
| *Do you lose urine for no reason at all?* | Pierde usted orina sin razón alguna? | **Pee-ehr**-deh oos-**tehd** oh-**ree**-nah seen rah-**sohn** ahl-**goo**-nah? |

| | | |
|---|---|---|
| Have you noticed a discharge from your penis? | Ha notado supuración de su pene? | Ah noh-**tah**-doh soo-poo-rah-**see**-**ohn** deh soo **peh**-neh? |
| Does your urine seem to have: | Parece que su orina tiene: | Pah-**reh**-seh keh soo oh-**ree**-nah **tee**-**eh**-neh: |
| * gas bubbles? | * burbujas de gas? | * boor-**boo**-hahs deh gahs? |
| * pus? | * pus? | * poos? |
| * solid particles? | * partículas solidas? | * pahr-**tee**-koo-lahs **soh**-lee-dahs? |
| Do you wait a long time for the urine to come out? | Espera mucho tiempo para que le salga la orina? | Ehs-**peh**-rah ■oo-choh tee-**ehm**-poh **pah**-rah keh leh **sahl**-gah lah oh-**ree**-nah? |
| Do you strain for the urine to come out? | Hace fuerza para que le salga la orina? | **Ah**-seh **fwehr**-sah **pah**-rah keh leh **sahl**-gah lah oh-**ree**-nah? |
| Does the urine take a long time to stop? | Se tarda mucho la orina en parar? | Seh **tahr**-dah ■oo-choh lah oh-**ree**-nah ehn pah-**rahr**? |
| Have you ever had: | Ha tenido alguna vez: | Ah teh-**nee**-doh ahl-**goo**-nah vehs: |
| * a bladder infection? | * una infección en la vejiga? | * **oo**-nah een-feg-**see**-**ohn** ehn lah veh-**hee**-gah? |
| * cystitis? | * cistitis? | * sees-**tee**-tees? |
| * kidney infection? | * infección de los riñones? | * een-feg-**see**-**ohn** deh lohs ree-**nyoh**-nehs? |
| * kidney stones? | * piedras en los riñones? | * **pee**-**eh**-drahs ehn lohs ree-**nyoh**-nehs? |
| * gallstone? | * piedras en la vesícula? | * **pee**-**eh**-drahs ehn lah veh-**see**-koo-lah? |
| * prostatitis? | * inflamación del próstata? | * een-flah-mah-**see**-**ohn** dehl **prohs**-tah-tah? |
| I have to examine you internally. | Tengo que examinarle internamente. | **Tehn**-goh keh eg-sah-mee-**nahr**-leh een-**tehr**-nah-■ehn-teh. |

Sexual history:

| | | |
|---|---|---|
| Have you ever had: | Alguna vez ha tenido: | Ahl-**goo**-nah vehs ah teh-**nee**-doh: |

50

| * Gonorrhea? | * Gonorrea? | * Goh-noh-**rheh-ah**? |
| * Herpes? | * Herpes? | * **Hehr**-pehs? |
| * Syphilis? | * Sífilis? | * **See**-fee-lees? |
| *Did you see a doctor?* | Vió al doctor? | Vee-**oh** ahl duck-**tohr**? |
| *Did you get penicillin?* | Le recetó penicilina? | Leh reh-seh-**toh** peh-nee-see-**lee**-nah? |
| *Did it get better?* | Se mejoró? | Seh meh-hoh-**roh**? |
| *How long ago were you ill?* | Cuánto tiempo estuvo enfermo? | **Kwahn**-toh tee-**ehm**-poh ehs-**too**-voh ehn-**fehr**-moh? |
| *Do you have any aches in your:* | Tiene algun dolor en sus: | **Tee-eh**-neh ahl-**goon** doh-**lohr** ehn soos: |
| * ankles? | * tobillos? | * toh-**bee**-yohs? |
| * joints? | * cojunturas? | * koh-yoon-**too**-rahs? |
| * knees? | * rodillas? | * roh-**dee**-yahs? |
| * wrists? | * muñecas? | * moo-**nyeh**-kahs? |
| *Have you had:* | Ha tenido usted: | Ah teh-**nee**-doh oos-**tehd**: |
| * a rash? | * salpullido? | * sahl-poo-**yee**-doh? |
| * fever? | * fiebre? | * **fee-eh**-breh? |
| * chills? | * escalofrios? | * ehs-kah-loh-**free-ohs**? |
| *Have you had any sores on your vagina?* | Ha tenido llagas/úlceras en su vagina? | Ah teh-**nee**-doh **yah**-gas/**ool**-seh-rahs ehn soo vah-**hee**-nah? |
| *Do you suffer from pain in your testicles?* | Sufre usted de dolor en los testículos? | **Soo**-freh oos-**tehd** deh doh-**lohr** ehn lohs tehs-**tee**-koo-lohs? |
| *Do you get a discharge from your penis?* | Tiene usted secreción (supuración) del pene? | **Tee-eh**-neh oos-**tehd** seh-kreh-**see-ohn** (soo-poo-rah-**see-ohn**) dehl **peh**-neh? |
| *Do you have any problems with fertility?* | Tiene problemas de fecundidad (fertilidad)? | **Tee-eh**-neh proh-**bleh**-mahs deh feh-**koon**-dee-dad (**fehr**-tee-lee-dad)? |
| *Do you get early morning erections?* | Se levanta en las mañanas con erección? | Seh leh-**vahn**-tah ehn lahs mah-**nyah**-nahs kohn eh-reg-**see-ohn**? |

| Have you noticed nocturnal emission of semen? | Ha notado en las noches emisión del semen? | Ah noh-**tah**-doh ehn lahs noh-chehs eh-mee-**see-ohn** dehl seh-**mehn**? |
| Are you aroused when you look at a woman rehsother than your wife deh soo ehs- or girlfriend? | Se excita cuando ve otras mujeres ademas | Seh eg-**see**-tah **kwahn**-doh veh **oh**-trahs moo-**heh**-dh-dehe**mah**sa o novia? poh-sah oh noh-vee-ah? |
| Are you able to masturbate to an erection or climax? | Se puede masturbar hasta alcanzar una erección o punto culminante? | Seh **pweh**-deh **mahs**-toor-bahr **ahs**-tah ahl-kahn-**sahr** oo-nah eh-reg-**see-ohn** oh **poon**-toh kool-mee-**nahn**-teh? |
| You must go to the Public Health Clinic. **Poo**-blee-kah. | Necesita ir a la Pública.de Salud | Neh-seh-**see**-tah eer ah **lebdKlee**-nee-kah deh Sah- |
| You have: | Usted tiene: | Oos-**tehd tee-eh**-neh: |
| * Syphilis | * Sífilis | * **See**-fee-lees |
| * Gonorrhea | * Gonorrea | * Goh-noh-**rheh-ah** |
| * Herpes | * Herpes | * **Hehr**-pehs |
| Are you allergic to Penicillin or other antibiotics? | Es alérgico a la Penicilina u otros antibióticos? | Ehs ah-**lehr**-hee-koh ah lah Peh-nee-see-**lee**-nah oo oh-trohs ahn-tee-**bee-oh**-tee-kohs? |

Pelvic Examination:

| I am going to do a pelvic examination. | Voy a hacerle un examen pélvico. | Voy ah ah-**sehr**-leh oon eg-**sah**-mehn **pehl**-vee-koh. |
| Put your feet in these stirrups. | Ponga los pies en estos estribos. | **Pohn**-gah lohs pee-ehs ehn **ehs**-tohs ehs-**treeh**-bohs. |
| Slide down some more. | Muévase mas hacia el borde. | **Mweh**-vah-seh mahs **ah**-see-ah ehl **bohr**-deh. |
| Relax your legs. | Relaje sus piernas. | Reh-**lah**-heh soos **pee-ehr**-nahs. |
| This might be a little cold. | Esto puede ser un poco frio. | **Ehs**-toh **pweh**-deh sehr oon **poh**-koh **free-oh**. |
| This will not hurt | Esto no le va a doler. | **Ehs**-toh noh leh vah ah doh-**lehr**. |

| | | |
|---|---|---|
| *I'm taking a sample.* | Estoy tomando un espécimen. | Ehs-**toy** toh-**mahn**-doh oon ehs-**peh**-see-mehn. |
| *I will now examine you internally with my fingers.* | Le examinaré internamente con mis dedos. | Leh eg-sah-mee-nah-**reh** een-tehr-nah-**mehn**-teh kohn mees **deh**-dohs. |
| *I'm going to examine your rectum.* | Voy a examinarle su recto. | Voy ah eg-sah-mee-**nahr**-leh soo **reg**-toh. |
| *Relax, this will not hurt.* | Relájese. Esto no le va a doler. | Reh-**lah**-heh-seh. **Ehs**-toh noh leh vah ah doh-**lehr**. |
| *Relax.* | Relájese. | Reh-**lah**-heh-seh. |
| *I'm finished.* | Terminé. (Acabé.) | Tehr-mee-**neh**. (Ah-kah-**beh**.) |
| *You can get dressed now.* | Puede vestirse ahora. | **Pweh**-deh vehs-**teer**-seh ah-**oh**-rah. |

Female Menses:

| | | |
|---|---|---|
| *How old were you when you started menstruating (your period)?* | Que edad tenia cuando empezó la menstruación (regla)? | Keh eh-**dad** teh-**nee-ah** **kwahn**-doh ehm-peh-**soh** lah **mehns**-troo-ah-**see-ohn** (**reh**-gla)? |
| *Are your periods regular?* | Son sus periodos (reglas) regulares? | Sohn soos peh-**ree**-oh-dohs (**reh**-glahs) reh-goo-**lah**-rehs? |
| *Do you bleed excessively with your periods?* | Sangra excesivamente en sus reglas? | **Sahn**-grah eg-seh-**see**-vah-**mehn**-teh ehn soos **reh**-glahs? |
| *Do you get:* | Le coge: | Leh coge: |
| * menstrual cramps? | * dolores en el vientre? | * doh-**loh**-rehs ehn ehl **vee-ehn**-treh? |
| * hot flashes? | * fogón de calor? | * foh-**gohn** deh kah-**lohr**? |
| * spottiness? | * manchas de sangre? | * **mahn**-chahs deh **sahn**-greh? |
| * sweating? | * mucho sudor? | * **moo**-choh soo-**dohr**? |
| * vaginal discharge/ itch? | * secreción/picazón vaginal? | * seh-kreh-**see-ohn**/pee-kah-**sohn** vah-hee-**nahl**? |
| *Do you use any form of birth control?* | Usa alguna forma anticonceptiva? | **Oo**-sah ahl-**goo**-nah **fohr**-mah **ahn**-tee-kohn-sep-**tee**-vah? |

53

| Do you use: | Usa usted: | Oo-sah oos-tehd: |
|---|---|---|
| * cervical cap? | * capa cervical? | * kah-pah sehr-vee-kahl? |
| * condoms? | * condon (gomas)? | * kohn-dohn (goh-mahs)? |
| * diaphragm? | * diafragma? | * dee-ah-frag-mah? |
| * IUD? | * diapositivo intra-uterino? | * dee-ah-poh-see-tee-voh een-trah-oo-teh-ree-noh? |
| * pills? | * pastillas anti-conceptivas? | * pahs-tee-yhahs ahn-tee-kohn-sep-tee-vahs? |
| * rhythm method? | * método ritmico? | * meh-toh-doh reet-mee-koh? |
| * vaginal foam cream? | * crema vaginal de espuma? | * kreh-mah vah-hee-nahl deh ehs-poo-mah? |
| * vasectomy? | * vasectomia? | * vah-sehg-toh-mee-ah? |

Pregnancy:

| | | |
|---|---|---|
| When was your last period? | Cuando fué su último periodo (regla)? | Kwahn-doh fweh soo ool-tee-moh peh-ree-oh-doh (reh-glah)? |
| Show me on the calendar. | Enséñeme en el calendario. | Ehn-seh-nyeh-meh ehn ehl kah-lehn-dah-ree-oh. |
| You are pregnant. | Usted está embarazada. | Oos-tehd ehs-tah ehm-bah-rah-sah-dah. |
| Is this your first pregnancy? | Es éste su primer embarazo? | Ehs ehs-teh soo pree-mehr ehm-bah-rah-soh? |
| How many times have you been pregnant? cinta)? | Cuántas veces ha éshado embarazada sah-dah (ehn seen-tah)? | Kwahn-tahs veh-sehs ah ehs-tah-doh ehm-bah-rah- |
| Please show me with your fingers. | Por favor enséñeme con sus dedos. | Pohr fah-vohr ehn-seh-nyeh-meh kohn soos deh-dohs. |
| Have you had any: | Ha tenido algun: | Ah teh-nee-doh ahl-goon: |
| * miscarriage? | * malparto? | * mahl-pahr-toh? |
| * abortion? | * aborto voluntario? | * ah-bohr-toh voh-loon-tah-ree-oh? |
| * stillbirths? | * nacimiento de niño muerto? | * nah-see-mee-ehn-toh deh nee-nyoh mwehr-toh? |

| | muerto? | nee-nyoh mwehr-toh? |
|---|---|---|
| How many children do you now have? | Cuántos niños tiene ahora? | Kwahn-tohs nee-nyohs tee-eh-neh ah-oh-rah? |

Labor:

| | | |
|---|---|---|
| Have your labor pains started? | Le han empezado los dolores? | Leh ahn ehm-peh-sah-doh lohs doh-loh-rehs? |
| Have you counted the minutes in between pain? | Ha contado los minutos entre dolor? | Ah kohn-tah-doh lohs mee-noo-tohs ehn-treh doh-lohr? |
| How many minutes apart? | Cada cuantos minutos aparte son? | Kah-dah kwahn-tohs mee-noo-tohs ah-pahr-teh sohn? |
| Show me on your fingers. | Enséñeme con sus dedos. | Ehn-seh-nyeh-meh kohn soos deh-dohs. |
| Has your water bag broken? | Se le ha roto la fuente (bolsa de agua)? | Seh leh ah roh-toh lah fwehn-teh (bohl-sah deh ah-gwah)? |
| Have you had any vaginal bleeding? | Ha sangrado por la vagina? | Ah sahn-grah-doh pohr lah vah-hee-nah? |
| Have you used many sanitary pads? | Ha usado muchas toallas higiénicas? | Ah oo-sah-doh moo-chahs toh-ah-yhahs ee-hee-eh-nee-kahs? |
| Show me on your fingers how many. | Enséñeme con sus dedos cuantas ha usado. | Ehn-seh-nyeh-meh kohn soos deh-dohs kwahn-tahs ah oo-sah-doh. |
| Do you have: | Tiene usted: | Tee-eh-neh oos-tehd: |
| * a headache | * dolor de cabeza? | * doh-lohr deh kah-beh-sah? |
| * swelling of the ankles? | * hinchazón de los tobillos? | * een-chah-sohn deh lohs toh-bee-yohs? |
| * vomiting? | * vomitos? | * voh-mee-tohs? |
| * dizziness? | * mareos? | * mah-reh-ohs? |

Delivery:

| | | |
|---|---|---|
| Are you having a: natural delivery? | Va a tener un parto natural? | Vah ah teh-nehr oon pahr-toh nah-too-rahl? |
| Let me check for dilatation. | Déjeme ver como está de dilatada. | Deh-heh-meh vehr koh-moh ehs-tah deh dee-lah-tah- |

55

dah.

| English | Spanish | Pronunciation |
|---|---|---|
| You are ready for delivery. | Está lista para el parto. | Ehs-**tah** **lees**-tah **pah**-rah ehl **pahr**-toh. |
| The nurse will get you ready. | La enfermera la preparará. | Lah ehn-fehr-**meh**-rah lah preh-pah-rah-**rah**. |
| Put your feet up in the stirrups. | Ponga los pies en estos estribos. | **Pohn**-gah lohs pee-ehs ehn **ehs**-tohs ehs-**tree**-bohs. |
| Spread your legs and knees apart. | Abra sus rodillas y piernas. | **Ah**-brah soos roh-**dee**-yahs ee **pee-ehr**-nahs. |
| Only push when I tell you. | Empúje sólo cuando le digo. | Ehm-**poo**-heh **soh**-loh **kwahn**-doh leh **dee**-goh. |
| Breathe in, and push. | Respire profundo y empúje. | Rehs-**pee**-reh proh-**foon**-doh ee ehm-**poo**-heh. |
| The baby is in the breech position. | El bebé está en posición de nalgas. | Ehl beh-**beh** ehs-**tah** ehn poh-see-**see-ohn** deh **nahl**-gas. |
| We have to do a cesarian. | Tenémos que hacer una cesárea. | Teh-**neh**-mohs keh ah-**sehr** **oo**-nah seh-**sah**-reh-ah. |

Endocrine:

| English | Spanish | Pronunciation |
|---|---|---|
| Have you ever had a thyroid problem? | Ha tenido problemas del tiroide? | Ah teh-**nee**-doh proh-**bleh**-mahs dehl tee-**roy**-deh? |
| Were you ever given medication for a thyroid trouble? | Le dieron medicina para el problema del tiroide? | Leh **dee-eh**-rohn meh-dee-**see**-nah **pah**-rah ehl proh-**bleh**-mah dehl tee-**roy**-deh? |
| Do you have: | Tiene usted: | **Tee-eh**-neh oos-**tehd**: |
| * a change in skin color? | * cambio de color en la piel? | * **kahm**-bee-oh deh koh-**lohr** ehn lah pee-ehl? |
| * anxiety/ agitation? | * ansiedad/ agitacion? | * ahn-see-eh-**dad**/ ah-**hee**-tah-**see-ohn**? |
| * cold intolerance? | * intolerancia al frio? | * **een**-toh-leh-**rahn**-see-ah ahl **free**-oh? |
| * diarrhea? | * diarrea? | * dee-ah-**rheh**-ah? |
| * excessive sweating? | * sudor excesivo? | * **soo**-dohr eg-seh-**see**-voh? |
| * heat intolerance? | * intolerancia al calor? | * een-toh-leh**rahn**-see-ah ahl kah-**lohr**? |

| English | Spanish | Pronunciation |
|---|---|---|
| * hoarseness? | * ronquera? | * rohn-**keh**-rah? |
| * insomnia? | * insomnia? | * een-**some**-nee-ah? |
| * loss of hair? | * pérdida de pelo? | * **pehr**-dee-dah deh **peh**-loh? |
| * palpitations? | * palpitaciones? | * pahl-pee-tah-**see-oh**-nehs? |
| * shakiness/ tremor? | * temblores/ tremores? | * tehm-**bloh**-rehs/ treh-**moh**-rehs? |
| * thick or enlarged tongue? | * lengua gruesa o alargada? | * **lehn**-gwah **grweh**-sah oh ah-lahr-**gah**-dah? |
| * weight loss despite good appetite? | * pérdida de peso aún con buén apetito? | * **pehr**-dee-dah deh **peh**-soh ah-**oon** kohn bwehn ah-peh-**tee**-toh? |
| *Do you have any lumps or bumps anywhere in your body?* | Tiene algún chichón o masas en su cuerpo? | **Tee-eh**-neh ahl-**goon** chee-**chohn** oh **mah**-sahs ehn soo **kwehr**-poh? |
| *Please show me where?* | Por favor, enséñeme adonde. | Pohr fah-**vohr** ehn-**seh**-nyeh-meh ah-**dohn**-deh. |
| *Has the lump changed in size?* | Ha cambiado la masa de tamaño? | Ah kahm-**bee-ah**-doh lah **mah**-sah deh tah-**mah**-nyoh? |

Extremities/Musculoskeletal:
Pain:

| English | Spanish | Pronunciation |
|---|---|---|
| *Did you get hurt by any of the following:* | Se dañó con uno de los siguientes: | Seh dah-**nyoh** kohn **oo**-noh deh lohs see-**gee-ehn**-tehs: |
| * fell down? | * se cayó? | * seh kah-**yhoh**? |
| * cut with a knife? | * se cortó con un cuchillo? | * seh kohr-**toh** kohn oon koo-**chee**-yhoh? |
| * shot with a gun? | * se pegó un balazo? | * seh peh-**goh** oon bah-**lah**-soh? |
| * in a car accident? | * en un acidente de carro? | * ehn oon ag-see-**dehn**-teh deh **kah**-rhoh? |
| * in another kind of accident? | * en otra clase de accidente? | * ehn **oh**-trah **klah**-seh deh ag-see-**dehn**-teh? |
| *Were you struck with an object?* | Fué golpeado con un objeto? | **Fweh** gohl-peh-**ah**-doh kohn oon ob-**heh**-toh? |

57

| Where do you feel the pain? | Donde siente el dolor? | **Dohn**-deh **see-ehn**-teh ehl doh-**lohr**? |
| Point to the spot that hurts the most. | Enséñeme con el dedo adonde le duele mas. | Ehn-**seh**-nyeh-meh kohn ehl **deh**-doh ah-**dohn**-deh leh **dweh**-leh mahs. |
| Do you get the pain daily? | Le coge el dolor diario? | Leh **koh**-heh ehl doh-**lohr** dee-**ah**-ree-oh? |
| Is the pain better in the: | Es mejor el dolor en la: | Ehs meh-**hohr** ehl doh-**lohr** ehn lah: |
| * morning? | * mañana? | * mah-**nyah**-nah? |
| * afternoon? | * tarde? | * **tahr**-deh? |
| * evening? | * noche? | * **noh**-cheh? |
| Does anything make the pain better/worse? | Hay algo que hace el dolor mejor/peor? | Ay **ahl**-goh keh **ah**-seh ehl doh-**lohr** meh-**hohr**/peh-ohr? |
| Do you take any medication to relieve the pain? | Toma alguna medicina para aliviar el dolor? | **Toh**-mah ahl-**goo**-nah meh-dee-**see**-nah **pah**-rah ah-lee-vee-ahr ehl doh-**lohr**? |
| Does the pain get better when you rest/exercise? | Se mejora el dolor si descansa o hace ejercicios? | Seh meh-**hoh**-rah ehl doh-**lohr** see dehs-**kahn**-sah oh **ah**-seh eh-**hehr**-see-see-ohs? |
| Does the pain change depending on the weather? | Le cambia el dolor de acuerdo al tiempo? | Leh **kahm**-bee-ah ehl doh-**lohr** deh ah-**kwehr**-doh ahl **tee-ehm**-poh? |
| Has the pain ever awaken you from sleep? | Lo ha despertado el dolor de dormir? | Loh ah dehs-pehr-**tah**-doh ehl doh-**lohr** deh dohr-**meer**? |
| Does the pain spread to other parts of the body? | Se extiende el dolor a otras partes del cuerpo? | Seh egs-**tee-ehn**-deh ehl doh-**lohr** ah **oh**-trahs **pahr**-tehs dehl **kwehr**-poh? |
| Does the pain change from one joint to another? | Cambia el dolor de una coyuntura a la otra? | **Kahm**-bee-ah ehl doh-**lohr** deh **oo**-nah koh-yoon-**too**-rah ah lah **oh**-trah? |
| Can you move your: | Puede mover su(s): | **Pweh**-deh moh-**vehr** soo(s): |
| * ankle(s)? | * tobillo(s)? | * toh-**bee**-yhoh(s)? |
| * back? | * espalda? | * ehs-**pahl**-dah? |

| English | Spanish | Pronunciation |
|---|---|---|
| * body? | * cuerpo? | * **kwehr**-poh? |
| * elbow(s)? | * codo(s)? | * **koh**-doh(s)? |
| * finger(s)? | * dedo(s)? | * **deh**-doh(s)? |
| * head? | * cabeza? | * kah-**beh**-sah? |
| * knee(s)? | * rodilla(s)? | * roh-**dee**-yhah(s)? |
| * leg(s)? | * pierna(s)? | * **pee**–**ehr**-nah(s)? |
| * toe(s)? | * dedo(s) del pie? | * **deh**-doh(s) dehl pee-eh? |
| * wrist(s)? | * muñeca(s)? | * moo-**nyeh**-kah(s)? |
| *Is your* _____ *weak?* | Tiene debil su: | **Tee**–**eh**-neh **deh**-beel soo: |
| * arm | * brazo? | * brah-soh? |
| * leg | * pierna? | * **pee**–**ehr**-nah? |
| * hand | * mano? | * **mah**-noh? |

| | | |
|---|---|---|
| *Have you recently had a sore throat?* | Reciéntemente ha tenido un dolor de garganta? | Reh-**see**–**ehn**-teh-**mehn**-teh ah teh-**nee**-doh oon doh-**lohr** deh gahr-**gahn**-tah? |
| *Please close your eyes.* | Por favor, cierre sus ojos. | Pohr fah-**vohr** see-**eh**-rheh soos **oh**-hohs. |
| *Do you feel this?* | Siente ésto? | **See**–**ehn**-teh **ehs**-toh? |
| *Is it sharp or dull?* | Lo siente puntiagudo o sin punto? | Loh **see**–**ehn**-teh **poon**-tee-ah-**goo**-doh oh seen **poon**-toh? |

## Posture Evaluation:

| | | |
|---|---|---|
| *Please, walk toward the wall on a straight line.* | Por favor, camine derecho hacia la pared. | Pohr fah-**vohr** kah-**mee**-neh deh-**reh**-choh **ah**-see-ah lah pah-**rehd**. |
| *Walk away from the wall on your tiptoes.* | Camine lejos de la pared en la punta de sus pies. | Kah-**mee**-neh **leh**-hohs deh lah pah-**rehd** ehn lah **poon**-tah deh soos pee-ehs. |
| *Walk on your heels.* | Camine en sus talones. | Kah-**mee**-neh ehn soos tah-**loh**-nehs. |

## Spine evaluation:

| | | |
|---|---|---|
| *Please bend:* | Por favor, dóblese hacia: | Pohr fah-**vohr**, **doh**-bleh-seh **ah**-see-ah: |

59

| | | |
|---|---|---|
| * backwards. | * atras. | * ah-**trahs**. |
| * forward. | * adelante. | * ah-deh-**lahn**-teh. |
| * to your right. | * su derecha. | * soo deh-**reh**-chah. |
| * to your left. | * su izquierda. | * soo ees-**kee-ehr**-dah. |

Neck rotation:

| | | |
|---|---|---|
| *Turn your head to the left.* | Volteé su cabeza a la izquierda. | Vol-**teh-eh** soo kah-**beh**-sah ah lah ees-**kee-ehr**-dah. |
| *Now to the right.* | Ahora a la derecha. | Ah-**oh**-rah ah lah deh-**reh**-chah. |
| *Touch your chin to your right shoulder.* | Tóque su hombro derecho con su barbilla. | **Toh**-keh soo **ohm**-broh deh-**reh**-choh kohn soo bar-**bee**-yhah. |
| *Now your left shoulder.* | Ahora su hombro izquierdo. | Ah-**oh**-rah soo **ohm**-broh ees-**kee-ehr**-doh. |
| *You have a:* | Usted tiene un: | Oos-**tehd tee-eh**-neh oon: |
| * broken bone. | * hueso quebrado. | * **hweh**-soh keh-**brah**-doh. |
| * sprained ankle. | * tobillo torcido. | * toh-**bee**-yhoh tohr-**see**-doh. |
| * dislocated shoulder. | * hombro dislocado. | * **ohm**-broh dees-loh-**kah**-doh. |
| * pulled muscle. | * músculo zafado. | * **moos**-koo-loh sah-**fah**-doh. |
| *You will need a:* | Necesita que se le ponga un: | Neh-seh-**see**-tah keh seh leh **pohn**-gah oon: |
| * cast. | * yeso. | * **jeh**-soh. |
| * dressing. | * vendaje. | * vehn-**dah**-heh. |
| * sling. | * cabestrillo. | * kah-behs-**tree**-yoh. |
| *Return immediately if your toes (fingers) get numb or blue.* | Regrese de inmediato si los dedos se entumecen o ponen azúl. | Reh-**greh**-seh deh **een**-meh-dee-**ah**-toh see lohs **deh**-dohs seh ehn-too-**meh**-sehn oh **poh**-nehn ah-**sool**. |
| *You need to rest in bed for _____:* (for numbers see Appendix 1) | Necesita estar en cama por _____: | Neh-seh-**see**-tah ehs-**tahr** ehn **kah**-mah pohr _____: |

60

| | | |
|---|---|---|
| * day(s). | * día(s). | * **dee**-ah(s). |
| * week(s). | * semana(s). | * seh-**mah**-nah(s). |
| * month(s) | * mes(es). | * **mehs**(es). |
| I will give you some pills for the pain. | Le daré unas pastillas para el dolor. | Leh dah-**reh** **oo**-nahs pahs-**tee**-yhahs **pah**-rah ehl doh-**lohr**. |
| Have you noticed any swelling on your: | Ha notado alguna hinchazón en sus: | Ah noh-**tah**-doh ahl-**goo**-nah **een**-chah-**sohn** ehn soos: |
| * joints? | * coyunturas? | * koh-yoon-**too**-rahs? |
| * muscles? | * músculos? | * **moos**-koo-lohs? |
| * other bones? | * otros huesos? | * **oh**-trohs **weh**-sohs? |
| Does Aspirin help? | Le ayuda la Aspirina? | Leh ah-**you**-dah lah Ahs-pee-**ree**-nah? |
| Do you experience any difficulty: | Tiene dificultad alguna: | **Tee-eh**-neh dee-fee-**kool**-tad ahl-**goo**-nah: |
| * dressing yourself? | * vistiéndose? | * vees-tee-**ehn**-doh-seh? |
| * combing your hair? | * peinándose? | * pay-**nahn**-doh-seh? |
| * holding a pen or pencil? | * agarrándo un lápiz? | * ah-gah-**rhahn**-doh oon **lah**-pees? |
| * lifting objects? | * levantándo objetos? | * leh-vahn-**tahn**-doh ob-**heh**-tohs? |
| * putting on your shoes? | * poniéndose los zapátos? | * poh-**nee-ehn**-doh-seh lohs sah-**pah**-tohs? |
| * sitting in a chair? | * sentándose en una silla? | * sehn-**tahn**-doh-seh ehn **oo**-nah see-yhah? |
| * standing in a chair? | * parándose en una silla? | * pah-**rahn**-doh-seh ehn **oo**-nah see-yhah? |
| * turning doorknobs? | * volteándo el picaporte (pomo de la puerta)? | * vohl-teh-**ahn**-doh ehl **pee**-kah-**pohr**-teh (**poh**-moh deh lah **pwehr**-tah)? |
| Are your muscles getting stiff? | Se le están poniendo los músculos rígidos? | Seh leh ehs-**tahn** poh-**nee-ehn**-doh lohs **moos**-koo-lohs **ree**-hee-dohs? |
| Have you noticed a | Ha notado disminución | Ah noh-**tah**-doh **dees**-mee- |

61

| decrease in: | en: | noo-**see-ohn** ehn: |
|---|---|---|
| * muscle size? | * el tamaño del músculo? | * ehl tah-**mah**-nyoh dehl **moos**-koo-loh? |
| * muscle strength? | * la fuerza del músculo? | * lah **fwerh**-sah dehl **moos**-koo-loh? |
| Is there a change in weakness as the day goes on? | Hay cambio de debilidad mientras pasa el día? | Ay **kahm**-bee-oh deh **deh**-bee-lee-dad **mee-ehn**-trahs **pah**-sah ehl **dee**-ah? |
| Does it get better or worse? | Se mejóra o empeóra? | Seh meh-**hoh**-rah oh ehm-peh-**oh**-rah? |
| Was the deformity gradual or suddenly? | Fué la deformidad gradual o repentina? | **Fweh** lah deh-**fohr**-mee-dad grah-**dwahl** oh reh-pehn-**tee**-nah? |
| How many ____ ago did you first notice it? | Hace cuántos ____ lo notó por primera ves? | **Ah**-seh **kwahn**-tohs ____ loh noh-**toh** pohr pree-**meh**-rah vehs: |
| * days? | * días? | * **dee**-ahs? |
| * weeks? | * semanas? | * seh-**mah**-nahs? |
| * months? | * meses? | * **meh**-sehs? |
| * years? | * años? | * **ah**-nyohs? |
| Is the deformity a result of a trauma? | Tiene la deformidad a causa de un trauma? | **Tee-eh**-neh lah deh-**fohr**-mee-dad ah **kah**-oo-sah deh oon **trah**-oo-mah? |
| Has the deformity changed with time? | Ha cambiado la deformidad con el tiempo? | Ah kahm-**bee-ah**-doh lah deh-**fohr**-mee-dad kohn ehl **tee-ehm**-poh? |
| Have you lost any feeling or strength in any part of your body? | Ha perdido algo de sensación o fuerza en alguna parte del cuerpo? | Ah per-**dee**-doh **ahl**-goh deh sehn-sah-**see-ohn** oh **fwehr**-sah ehn ahl-**goo**-nah **pahr**-teh dehl **kwehr**-poh? |
| Was any part of your body ever paralyzed? | Fué paralizada alguna parte de su cuerpo? | Fweh **pah**-rah-lee-**sah**-dah ahl-**goo**-nah **pahr**-teh deh soo **kwehr**-poh? |
| What did you first notice: | Que notó por primera ves: | Keh noh-**toh** pohr pree-**meh**-rah vehs: |
| * a lump? | * el chichón? | * ehl chee-**chohn**? |
| * pain? | * el dolor? | * ehl doh-**lohr**? |

| | | |
|---|---|---|
| * paralysis? | * la parálisis? | * lah pah-**rah**-lee-sees? |
| * weakness? | * la debilidad? | * lah **deh**-bee-lee-dad? |
| *Was it very painful?* | Fué muy doloroso? | **Fweh** mooy doh-loh-**roh**-soh? |
| *Has the lump changed in size?* | Ha cambiado de tamaño el chichón? | Ah kahm-bee-**ah**-doh deh tah-**mah**-nyoh ehl chee-**chohn**? |
| *Are you constantly tired or exhausted?* | Está cansado o agotádo constantemente? | Ehs-**tah** kahn-**sah**-doh oh ah-goh-**tah**-doh kohns-tahn-teh-**mehn**-teh? |

Neurological:

| | | |
|---|---|---|
| *I would like to ask you some questions.* | Me gustaría hacerle unas preguntas. | Meh goos-tah-**ree-ah** ah-**sehr**-leh **oo**-nahs preh-**goon**-tahs? |
| *What is your name?* | Cuál es su nombre? | Kwahl ehs soo **nohm**-breh? |
| *What date is it?* | Que fecha es hoy? | Keh **feh**-chah ehs oy? |
| *Please tell me the day of the week.* | Por favor dígame que día de la semana es? | Pohr fah-**vohr dee**-gah-meh keh **dee**-ah deh lah seh-**mah**-nah ehs? |
| *Where are we now?* | Dónde estamos ahora? | **Dohn**-deh ehs-**tah**-mohs ah-**oh**-rah? |
| *Repeat after me: no if, ands or buts.* | Repita despues de mi: no, si, ys o pero. | Reh-**pee**-tah dehs-**pwehs** deh mee: noh, see, ees, oh **peh**-roh. |
| *Have you ever lost consciousness before?* | Ha perdido el conocimiento alguna vez? | Ah pehr-**dee**-doh ehl koh-noh-see-**mee-ehn**-toh ahl-**goo**-nah vehs? |
| *Did anyone see it happen?* | Alguién vió lo que pasó? | Ahl-**gee-ehn** vee-**oh** loh keh pah-**soh**? |
| *Did you have a warning prior to the attack?* | Sintió como un aviso antes del atáque? | Seen-**tee-oh koh**-moh oon ah-**vee**-soh **ahn**-tehs dehl ah-**tah**-keh? |
| *Were you told of any body movements?* | Le dijerón de algún movimiento en el cuerpo? | Leh dee-**heh**-rohn deh ahl-**goon** moh-vee-**mee-ehn**-toh ehn ehl **kwehr**-poh? |
| *Was there a period of sleepiness following the attack?* | Se quedó dormido despues del atáque? | Seh keh-**doh** dohr-**mee**-doh dehs-**pwehs** dehl ah-**tah**-keh? |
| *Did you feel confused* | Se sintió confundido | Seh seen-**tee-oh** kohn- |

63

| afterwards? | despues? | foon-**dee**-doh dehs-**pwehs**? |
|---|---|---|
| *Was there any loss of* urine or bowel control during the attack? | Perdió el control de la orina y feces durante el atáque? | Pehr-**dee-oh** ehl kohn-**trohl** deh lah oh-**reen**-nah ee **feh**-ses doo-**rahn**-teh ehl ah-**tah**-keh? |
| *Is your memory clear* for what happened just before the attack? | Se acuerda bien de lo que pasó antes del atáque? | Seh ah-**kwehr**-dah **bee-ehn** deh loh keh pah-**soh ahn**-tehs dehl ah-**tah**-keh? |
| *Do you suffer from:* | Sufre usted de: | **Soo**-freh oos-**tehd** deh: |
| * clumsiness? | * falta de destreza? | * **fahl**-tah deh dehs-**treh**-sah? |
| * dizziness? | * mareos? | * mah-**reh**-ohs? |
| * staggering? | * tambaleo? | * tahm-bah-**leh-oh**? |
| * unsteady gait? | * falta de coordinacion? | * **fahl**-tah deh koh-ohr-dee-nah-**see-ohn**? |
| *Have you ever had:* | Ha tenido usted: | Ah teh-**nee**-doh oos-**tehd**: |
| * seizures? | * atáques epilépticos? | * ah-**tah**-kehs eh-pee-**lep**-tee-kohs? |
| * convulsions? | * convulsiones? | * kohn-vool-see-**oh**-nehs? |
| * fainting or fainting spells? | * desmayos o desvanecimientos? | * dehs-**mah**-yhohs oh **des**-vah-neh-see-**mee-ehn**-tohs? |
| *Is your dizziness* worse with your eyes opened or closed? | Es su maréo peor con los ojos cerrados o abiertos? | Ehs soo mah-**reh**-oh peh-**ohr** kohn lohs oh-**hohs** seh-**rhah**-dohs oh ah-**bee-ehr**-tohs? |
| *Do you get a pain in* your hip or leg when walking? | Le coge dolor en la pierna o cadera cuando camina? | Leh **koh**-heh doh-**lohr** ehn lah **pee-ehr**-nah oh kah-**deh**-rah **kwahn**-doh kah-**mee**-nah? |
| *Do you have any* problems with: | Tiene problemas con: | **Tee-eh**-neh proh-**bleh**-mahs kohn: |
| * ejaculation? | * eyaculación? | * **eh**-yhah-koo-lah-**see-ohn**? |
| * an erection? | * erección? | * eh-reg-**see-ohn**? |
| *Is there a history* of diabetes? | Tiene historial de diabetes? | **Tee-eh**-neh ees-**toh**-ree-ahl deh dee-ah-**beh**-tehs? |

| | | |
|---|---|---|
| *Do you use any of the following:* | Usa alguno de los siguientes: | **Oo**-sah ahl-**goo**-noh deh lohs see-**gee**-**ehn**-tehs: |
| * alcohol? | * alcohol/licor? | * ahl-**kohl**/lee-**kohr**? |
| * depressants? | * depresantes? | * deh-preh-**sahn**-tehs? |
| * insulin? | * insulina? | * **een**-soo-**lee**-nah? |
| * street drugs? | * drogas de calle? | * **droh**-gahs deh **kah**-yheh? |
| *Have you ever had an injury to your head?* | Ha sufrido algun daño a la cabeza? | Ah soo-**free**-doh ahl-**goon** dah-nyoh ah lah kah-**beh**-sah? |
| *Have you noticed a change in your speech pattern?* | Ha notado algún cambio en su forma de hablar? | Ah noh-**tah**-doh ahl-**goon** **kahm**-bee-oh ehn soo **fohr**-mah deh ah-**blahr**? |
| *Is your speech thick or slurred?* | Es su forma de hablar poco clara o incomprensible? | Ehs soo **fohr**-mah deh ah-**blahr** poh-koh **klah**-rah oh een-kohm-prehn-**see**-bleh? |
| *Do you understand things said to you?* | Entiénde las cosas que le dicen? | Ehn-**tee**-**ehn**-deh lahs **koh**-sahs keh leh **dee**-sehn? |
| *Has there been a change in your handwriting?* | Ha habido algún cambio en su forma de escribir? | Ah ah-**bee**-doh ahl-**goon** **kahm**-bee-oh ehn soo **fohr**-mah deh ehs-kree-**beehr**? |
| *Is your memory worse lately?* | Esta su memoria peor ultimamente? | Ehs-**tah** soo meh-**moh**-ree-ah peh-**ohr** ool-tee-mah-**mehn**-teh? |

**To the Relatives:**

| | | |
|---|---|---|
| *Has the patient's behavior changed lately?* | Ha cambiado el comportamiento del paciente últimamente? | Ah kahm-**bee**-**ah**-doh ehl kohm-**pohr**-tah-**mee**-**ehn**-toh dehl pah-**see**-**ehn**-teh ool-tee-mah-**mehn**-teh? |
| *Did the patient stop:* | Dejó el paciente de: | Deh-**hoh** ehl pah-**see**-**ehn**-teh deh: |
| * eating? | * comer? | * koh-**mehr**? |
| * sleeping? | * dormir? | * dohr-**meehr**? |
| * speaking? | * hablar? | * ah-**blahr**? |
| *Does the patient use:* | Usa el paciente: | **Oo**-sah ehl pah-**see**-**ehn**-teh: |
| * alcohol? | * alcohol (licor)? | * ahl-**kohl** (lee-**kohr**)? |

| * street drugs? | * drogas de calle? | * **droh**-gahs deh **kah**-yheh? |
|---|---|---|
| *Has the patient* become withdrawn? | Se volvió el paciente remoto/retirado? | Seh vohl-**vee-oh** ehl pah-**see-ehn**-teh reh-**moh**-toh/ reh-tee-**rah**-doh? |

<u>Motor Functioning</u>:

| *Sit here facing me.* | Siéntese aqui en frente de mi. | **See-ehn**-teh-seh ah-**kee** ehn-**frehn**-teh deh mee. |
|---|---|---|

<u>Finger to nose test</u>:

| *Please close your eyes* and touch your nose with your index finger. | Por favor cierre sus ojos y toque su nariz con su dedo índice. | Pohr fah-**vohr** see-**eh**-rreh soos oh-**hohs** ee toh-keh soo nah-**reehs** kohn soo **deh**-doh **een**-dee-seh. |
|---|---|---|
| *Now use the other* hand. | Ahora use la otra mano. | Ah-**oh**-rah **oo**-seh lah **oh**-trah **mah**-noh. |

<u>Test flexion/extension of arm</u>:

| *Push down your arm and* don't let me pull it up. | Empúje su brazo hacia abajo y no deje que yo lo suba. | Ehm-**poo**-heh soo **brah**-soh **ah**-see-ah ah-**bah**-hoh ee noh **deh**-heh keh yhoh loh **soo**-bah. |
|---|---|---|
| *Pull up your arm and* don't let me push it down. | Levante su brazo hacia arriba y no deje que yo lo empuje. | Leh-**vahn**-teh soo **brah**-soh **ah**-see-ah ah-**ree**-bah ee noh **deh**-heh keh yhoh loh ehm-**poo**-heh. |

<u>Patellar Tendon Reflex Text</u>:

| *Let your legs dangle* down. | Deje que sus piernas le cuelgen. | **Deh**-heh keh soos **pee-ehr**-nahs leh **kwehl**-gehn. |
|---|---|---|
| *Relax.* | Relájese. | Reh-**lah**-heh-seh. |
| *I will strike your* knee with this reflex hammer. | Voy a examinar el reflejo de su rodilla con esto. | Voy ah **eg**-sah-mee-**nahr** ehl reh-**fleh**-hoh deh soo roh-**dee**-yah kohn **ehs**-toh. |
| *You have had this done* before, haven't you? | A usted le han hecho esto antes, no? | Ah oos-**tehd** leh ahn **eh**-choh **ehs**-toh **ahn**-tehs, noh? |
| It won't hurt you. | No le va a doler. | Noh leh vah ah doh-**lehr**. |

<u>Test pain sensation</u>:

| *This is a needle which* I'm going to use to test your foot. | Voy a usar esta aguja para probar su sensa- ción del pié. | Voy ah oo-**sahr ehs**-tah ah-**goo**-hah **pah**-rah proh-**bahr** soo sehn-sah-**see-ohn** |
|---|---|---|

dehl pee-eh.

| English | Spanish | Pronunciation |
|---|---|---|
| *Please close your eyes and tell me if you feel it.* | Por favor cierre sus ojos y dígame si lo siente. | Pohr fah-**vohr** see-**eh**-rheh soos oh-**hohs** ee dee-**gah**-meh see loh see-**ehn**-teh. |
| *Can you feel this?* | Siente esto? | See-**ehn**-teh ehs-toh? |
| *Is this sharp?* | Lo siente puntiagudo? | Loh see-**ehn**-teh poon-tee-ah-**goo**-doh? |
| *Is this dull?* | Lo siente sin punta? | Loh see-**ehn**-teh seen poon-tah? |

## Evaluation of external rotation of arm:

| English | Spanish | Pronunciation |
|---|---|---|
| *Stretch out your arms with your fingers spread.* | Extienda sus brazos con sus dedos abiertos. | Egs-**tee-ehn**-dah soos **brah**-sohs kohn soos **deh**-dohs ah-**bee-ehr**-tohs. |
| *Extend your arms fully and place your palms together above your head.* | Extienda sus brazos arriba de su cabeza con las palmas juntas. | Egs-**tee-ehn**-dah soos **brah**-sohs ah-**rhee**-bah deh soo kah-**beh**-sah kohn lahs **pahl**-mahs **hoon**-tahs. |
| *Place your hands on your back.* | Ponga sus manos en su espalda. | **Pohn**-gah soos ■ah-nohs ehn soo ehs **pahl**-dah. |
| *Like this.* (Show how) | Así como esto. | Ah-**see koh**-moh ehs-toh. |

## Assessing strenght of upper extremities:

| English | Spanish | Pronunciation |
|---|---|---|
| *Hold these two fingers of my hands and resist any movement from me.* | Agarre mis dedos y resista cualquier movimiento. | Ah-**gah**-rheh mees **deh**-dohs ee reh-**sees**-tah kwahl-**kee-ehr** moh-vee-■ee-ehn-toh. |
| *Please lie down, I'll now lift up your leg.* | Por favor acuéstese, ahora le levanto su pierna. | Pohr fah-**vohr** ah-**kwehs**-teh-seh, ah-**oh**-rah leh leh-**vahn**-toh soo pee-**ehr**-nah. |
| *Can you flex your foot: Up? Down?* | Puede doblar su pie: Hacia arriba? Hacia abajo? | **Pweh**-deh doh-**blahr** soo **pee**-eh: **Ah**-see-ah ah-**rhee**-bah? **Ah**-see-ah ah-**bah**-hoh? |
| *Sit on the side of the bed and flex your neck, placing your chin on your chest.* | Siéntese al lado de la cama y ponga su barbilla en su pecho. | See-**ehn**-teh-seh ahl **lah**-doh deh lah **kah**-mah ee **pohn**-gah soo bahr-**bee**-yhah ehn soo **peh**-choh. |
| *Can you do this?* | Puede hacer esto? | **Pweh**-deh ah-**sehr** ehs-toh? |

67

## For Outpatients:

*Do you have a written order from your doctor?*

Tiene una orden escrita de su doctor?

**Tee-eh**-neh **oo**-nah **ohr**-dehn ehs-**kree**-tah deh soo duck-**tohr**?

*May I see your doctor's orders?*

Puedo ver las ordenes del doctor?

**Pweh**-doh vehr lahs **ohr**-deh-nehs dehl duck-**tohr**?

*Please give me your health insurance card.*

Por favor deme su tarjeta del seguro médico.

Pohr fah-**vohr deh**-meh soo tahr-**heh**-tah dehl seh-**goo**-roh **meh**-dee-koh.

*Please have a seat until your name is called.*

Por favor siéntese hasta que llamen su nombre.

Pohr fah-**vohr see-ehn**-teh-seh **ahs**-tah keh **yhah**-mehn soo **nohm**-breh.

*Did you have breakfast this morning?*

Desayunó esta mañana?

Deh-sah-you-**noh ehs**-tah mah-**nyah**-nah?

*You are not to eat anything after midnight.*

No puede comer nada despues de medianoche.

Noh **pweh**-deh koh-**mehr nah**-dah dehs-**pwehs** deh **meh**-dee-ah-**noh**-cheh.

*This test must be done on an empty stomach.*

Este análisis tiene que ser hecho con el estómago vacio.

**Ehs**-teh ah-**nah**-lee-sees **tee-eh**-neh keh sehr **eh**-choh kohn ehl ehs-**toh**-mah-goh vah-**see-oh**.

*You need to eat a good breakfast.*

Necesita comer un buen desayuno.

Neh-seh-**see**-tah koh-**mehr** oon bwehn deh-sah-**you**-noh.

## Venipuncture:

*I need to draw some blood from your arm.*

Necesito sacarle sangre del brazo.

Neh-seh-**see**-toh sah-**kahr**-leh **sahn**-greh dehl **brah**-soh.

*Have you had a blood test done before?*

Ha tenido un examen de sangre antes?

Ah teh-**nee**-doh oon eg-**sah**-meh deh **sahn**-greh **ahn**-tehs?

*This will hurt only a little bit.*

Esto va a dolerle sólo un poquito.

**Ehs**-toh vah ah doh-**lehr**-leh **soh**-loh oon poh-**kee**-toh.

*Please roll up your sleeve.*

Por favor súbase la manga.

Pohr fah-**vohr soo**-bah-seh lah **mahn**-gah.

*Stretch your arm out and make a fist.*

Extienda su brazo y haga un puño.

Egs-**tee-ehn**-dah soo **brah**-soh ee **ah**-gah oon **poo**-nyoh.

| English | Spanish | Pronunciation |
|---|---|---|
| That's good. | Asi está bièn. | Ah-**see** ehs-**tah** bee-ehn. |
| You will feel a small needle stick. | Sentirá un pequeño piquète. | Sehn-tee-**rah** oon peh-**keh**-nyoh pee-**keh**-teh. |
| Hold still. Open your hand slowly. | No se mueva. Abra su mano poco a poco. | Noh seh **mweh**-vah. **Ah**-brah soo **mah**-noh **poh**-koh ah **poh**-koh. |
| Hold this tight with your fingers. | Apriète esto duro con sus dedos. | Ah-**pree-eh**-teh **ehs**-toh **doo**-roh kohn soos **deh**-dohs. |
| Your veins are hard to find. | Sus venas son duras de encontrar. | Soos **veh**-nahs sohn **doo**-rahs deh **ehn**-kohn-trahr. |
| I need to get a few drops of blood from you finger. | Necesito sacar unas gotas de sangre de su dedo. | Neh-seh-**see**-toh sah-**kahr** **oo**-nahs **goh**-tahs deh **sahn**-greh deh soo **deh**-doh. |
| Hold the baby still. | No deje que se mueva el bebè. | Noh **deh**-heh keh seh **mweh**-vah ehl beh-**beh**. |
| I need a few drops of blood from your baby's heel. | Necesito unas gotas de sangre del talòn del bebè. | Neh-seh-**see**-toh **oo**-nahs **goh**-tahs deh **sahn**-greh dehl tah-**lohn** dehl beh-**beh**. |

Urine:

| English | Spanish | Pronunciation |
|---|---|---|
| Can you give me a sample of urine? | Puede darme una muestra de orina? | **Pweh**-deh **dahr**-meh **oo**-nah **mwehs**-trah deh oh-**ree**-nah? |
| Bring the urine specimen in this. | Traiga la muestra de orina en esto. | **Trah-ee**-gah lah **mwehs**-trah deh oh-**ree**-nah en **ehs**-toh. |

Instructions:

| English | Spanish | Pronunciation |
|---|---|---|
| First wipe off the urethra with this swab. | Primero limpiese con esto antes de coger la muestra. | Pree-**meh**-roh **lee**-pee-eh-seh kohn **ehs**-toh **ahn**-tehs deh koh-**hehr** lah **mwehs**-trah. |
| Then start urinating in the toilet. | Empiese a orinar en la taza del baño. | Ehm-**pee-eh**-seh ah oh-ree-**nahr** ehn lah **tah**-sah dehl **bah**-nyoh. |
| After a second or two, fill the container half full. | Despues de uno o dos segundos, llene este frasco a la mitad. | Dehs-**pwehs** deh **oo**-noh oh dohs seh-**goon**-dohs, **jeh**-neh **ehs**-teh **frahs**-koh ah lah mee-**tahd**. |

69

## Sputum:

| | | |
|---|---|---|
| *I need a specimen of* your phlegm/sputum after you cough. | Necesito una muestra de su flema/esputo cuando toce. | Neh-seh-**see**-toh **oo**-nah **mwehs**-trah deh soo **fleh**-mah/ehs-**poo**-toh **kwahn**-doh **toh**-seh. |
| *Take this and use it* for phlegm/sputum. | Llévese esto y úselo para su flema/esputo. | **Jeh**-veh-seh **ehs**-toh ee **oo**-seh-loh **pah**-rah soo **fleh**-mah/ehs-**poo**-toh. |
| Remember to cough deeply. I don't want saliva. | Recuerde de tocer profundo. No quiero saliva. | Reh-**kwehr**-deh deh toh-**sehr** proh-**foon**-doh. Noh **kee-eh**-roh sah-**lee**-vah. |

## Stool:

| | | |
|---|---|---|
| *Please, take this* laxative tonight. | Por favor, tome este purgante esta noche. | Pohr fah-**vohr** **toh**-meh **ehs**-teh poor-**gahn**-teh **ehs**-tah **noh**-cheh. |
| *Bring a stool* specimen tomorrow. | Traiga una muestra de su excremento mañana. | **Trah-ee**-gah **oo**-nah **mwehs**-trah deh soo egs-kreh-**mehn**-toh mah-**nyah**-nah. |

## Throat Culture:

| | | |
|---|---|---|
| *Open your mouth,* please | Abra su boca, por favor. | **Ah**-brah soo **boh**-kah pohr fah-**vohr**. |
| *I'm going to swab your* tonsils and throat with this cotton end. | Le voy a frotar las anginas/amigdalas con éste algodón. | Leh voy ah froh-**tahr** lahs ahn-**hee**-nahs/ah-**meeg**-dah-lahs kohn **ehs**-teh ahl-goh-**dohn**. |
| *It is normal to feel* like you want to gag. | Es normal que se sienta como que se atraganta. | Ehs norh-**mahl** keh seh **see-ehn**-tah **koh**-moh keh seh ah-trah-**gahn**-tah. |
| *We'll know the results* in the next 24 hours. | Sabrémos los resultados en veinticuatro horas. | Sah-**breh**-mohs lohs reh-sool-**tah**-dohs ehn vain-tee-**kwah**-troh **oh**-rahs. |
| *We will call and let* you know if it is positive. | Le llamaremos para darle a saber si es positivo. | Leh yhah-mah-**reh**-mohs **pah**-rah **dahr**-leh ah sah-**behr** see ehs poh-see-**tee**-voh. |

## Electrocardiogram (ECG):

| | | |
|---|---|---|
| *Your doctor has* ordered an electrocardiogram. | Su doctor ha ordenado un electrocardiograma. | Soo **duck**-tohr ah ohr-deh-**nah**-doh oon eh-**leg**-troh-kar-dee-oh-**grah**-mah. |

70

| Is this your first ECG? | Es este su primer electrocardiograma? | Ehs **ehs**-teh soo pree-**mehr** eh-**leg**-troh-kar-dee-oh-**grah**-mah? |
|---|---|---|
| Is this your first ECG in this hospital? | Es este su primer electrocardiograma en este hospital? | Ehs **ehs**-teh soo pree-**mehr** eh-**leg**-troh-kar-dee-oh-**grah**-mah ehn **ehs**-teh ohs-pee-**tahl**? |
| Please, lie down in bed. | Por favor, acuéstese en la cama. | Pohr fah-**vohr** ah-**kwehs**-teh-seh ehn lah **kah**-mah. |
| Put your arms and legs down. | Ponga sus brazos y piernas rectas. | **Pohn**-gah soos **brah**-sohs ee **pee-ehr**-nahs reg-tahs. |
| Relax. Please don't move or speak during the test. | Relajese. Por favor no se mueva o hable durante el examen. | Reh-**lah**-heh-seh. Pohr fah-**vohr** noh seh **mweh**-vah oh **ah**-bleh doo-**rahn**-teh ehl eg-**sah**-mehn. |
| The test will only take a few minutes. | El examen tomará sólo unos minutos. | Ehl eg-**sah**-mehn toh-mah-**rah** soh-**loh** **oo**-nohs mee-**noo**-tohs. |
| This will not hurt. | Esto no va a dolerle. | **Ehs**-toh noh vah ah doh-**lehr**-leh. |

Radiology:

| Have you had x-rays done here before? | Le han tomado radio-grafías aquí antes? | Leh ahn toh-**mah**-doh rah-dee-oh-grah-**fee-ahs** ah-**kee ahn**-tehs? |
|---|---|---|
| Take your top off and put on this gown. | Quítese la ropa y póngase este camisón. | **Kee**-teh-seh lah **rhoh**-pah ee **pohn**-gah-seh **ehs**-teh kah-mee-**sohn**. |
| Remove your necklace if you have any on. | Quítese la cadena si lleva una puesta. | **Kee**-teh-seh lah kah-**deh**-nah see **jeh**-vah **oo**-nah **pwehs**-tah. |
| Stand here and place your shoulders and chest against this plate. | Párese aqui y ponga su pecho y hombros contra esta placa. | **Pah**-reh-seh ah-**kee** ee **pohn**-gah soo **peh**-choh ee **ohm**-brohs **kohn**-trah **ehs**-tah **plah**-kah. |
| Rest your chin here. | Ponga su barbilla aquí. | **Pohn**-gah soo **bar**-bee-yhah ah-**kee**. |
| Rest the back of your hands on your hips. | Ponga la parte trasera de sus manos en sus caderas. | **Pohn**-gah lah **pahr**-teh trah-**seh**-rah deh soos **mah**-nohs ehn soos kah-**deh**-rahs. |
| Don't move. | No se mueva. | Noh seh **mweh**-vah. |

| | | |
|---|---|---|
| *Take a deep breath.* Hold it. | Respire profundo y manténgalo. | Rhehs-**pee**-reh proh-**foon**-doh ee mahn-**tehn**-gah-loh. |
| *You may breathe.* | Puede respirar. | **Pweh**-deh rehs-pee-**rahr**. |
| *Turn to your right (left).* | Volteése al lado derecho (izquierdo). | Vol-**teh-eh**-seh ahl **lah**-doh deh-**reh**-choh (ees-**kee-ehr**-doh). |
| *Put your hands on top of your head.* | Ponga sus manos arriba de su cabeza. | **Pohn**-ah soos ■ah-nohs ah-**rhee**-bah deh soo kah-**beh**-sah. |
| *Please, lie on the table on your back/ stomach.* | Por favor, acuestese en la mesa en su espalda/estómago. | Pohr fah-**vohr** ah-**kwehs**-teh-seh ehn lah ■eh-sah ehn soo ehs-**pahl**-dah/ ehs-**toh**-mah-goh. |
| *Breathe in. Hold your breath. Breathe out.* | Respire profundo. Manténgalo. Respire normal. | Rehs-**pee**-reh proh-**foon**-doh. Mahn-**tehn**-gah-loh. Rehs-**pee**-reh nohr-■ahl. |
| *We are finished.* | Acabamos. | Ah-kah-**bah**-mohs. |
| *Sit down on a chair* outside to wait. | Siéntese afuera a esperar. | **See-ehn**-teh-seh ah-**fweh**-rah ah ehs-peh-**rahr**. |
| I have to see if they turned out. | Tengo que ver si salieron bien. | **Tehn**-goh keh vehr see sah-**lee-eh**-rohn bee-ehn. |
| *We need to repeat the* x-rays. | Necesito tomar las placas otra ves. | Neh-seh-**see**-toh toh-■ahr lahs **plah**-kahs **oh**-trah vehs. |
| *You may get dressed.* | Puede vestirse. | **Pweh**-deh vehs-**teer**-seh. |

Ultrasound:

| | | |
|---|---|---|
| *Please, undress and* put on this gown. | Por favor, quítese la ropa y póngase este camisón. | Pohr fah-**vohr kee**-teh-seh lah **rhoh**-pah ee **pohn**-gah- seh **ehs**-teh kah-mee-**sohn**. |
| *Did you drink water or* other liquids? | Tomó agua o algún otro líquido? | Toh-■oh ah-gwah oh ahl-**goon oh**-troh **lee**-kee-doh? |
| *Does your bladder* feel full? | Siente su vejiga llena? | **See-ehn**-teh soo veh-**hee**-gah **yheh**-nah? |
| *Your bladder needs to* be full for this test. | Su vejiga necesita estar llena para este examen. | Soo veh-**hee**-gah neh-seh-**see**-tah ehs-**tahr jeh**-nah **pah**-rah **ehs**-teh eg-**sah**-mehn. |

| English | Spanish | Pronunciation |
|---|---|---|
| Have you had an ultrasound done before? | Ha tenido un ultrasonido antes? | Ah teh-**nee**-doh oon **ool**-trah-soh-**nee**-doh **ahn**-tehs? |
| This test will not hurt you. | Este examen no le va a doler. | **Ehs**-teh eg-**sah**-mehn noh leh vah ah doh-**lehr**. |
| I will rub some mineral oil on your skin. | Voy a frotarle aceite mineral en su piel. | Voy ah froh-**tahr**-leh ah-**sey**-teh mee-neh-rahl ehn soo **pee-ehl**. |
| The sound goes into your body much better with some oil. | El sonido pasa mejor por su cuerpo con el aceite. | Ehl soh-**nee**-doh **pah**-sah meh-**hohr** pohr soo **kwehr**-poh kohn ehl ah-**sey**-teh. |

CT Scan:

| English | Spanish | Pronunciation |
|---|---|---|
| Take off your clothes and put on this gown. | Quítese la ropa y póngase este camisón. | **Kee**-teh-seh lah **rhoh**-pah ee **pohn**-gah-seh **ehs**-teh kah-mee-**sohn**. |
| Lie down on this table. | Acuéstese en la mesa. | Ah-**kwehs**-teh-seh ehn lah **meh**-sah. |
| I will move you in to the ring of the scanner. | Lo movere al círculo del contador. | Loh moh-veh-**reh** ahl **seer**-koo-loh dehl kohn-tah-**dohr**. |
| As I move you through the scanner, don't move. | Mientras lo muevo a traves del contador, no se mueva | **Mee-ehn**-trahs loh **mweh**-voh ah trah-**vehs** dehl kohn-tah-**dohr**, noh seh **mweh**-vah. |
| You will hear sounds of gear/motor as the x-ray scans your body. | Oirá ruidos de motor mientras el contador explora su cuerpo. | Oh-**eer**ah **rwee**-dohs deh moh-**tohr** **mee-ehn**-trahs ehl kohn-tah-**dohr** egs-**ploh**-rah soo **kwehr**-poh. |
| The table will move you in position for the next scan. | La mesa lo moverá de posición para la próxima imagen. | Lah **meh**-sah loh moh-**veh**-rah deh poh-see-**see-ohn** **pah**-rah lah **prog**-see-mah ee-mah-hen. |
| Relax. Remain as still as possible. | Relájese. Manténgase tan rígido como sea posible. | Reh-**lah**-heh-seh. Mahn-**tehn**-gah-seh tahn **ree**-hee-doh **koh**-moh leh seh-ah poh-**see**-bleh. |
| Hold your breath. Breathe again. | Aguante su respiración. Puede Respirar. | Ah-**gwahn**-teh soo **rehs**-pee-rah-**see-ohn**. **Pweh**-deh **rehs**-pee-rahr. |

Electroencephalogram (EEG):

| English | Spanish | Pronunciation |
|---|---|---|
| Wash your hair the | Lávese el pelo la | **Lah**-veh-seh ehl **peh**-loh |

| | | |
|---|---|---|
| night before. | noche antes. | lah **noh**-cheh **ahn**-tehs. |
| *Do not use any hair* *spray or gel.* | No use laca ni grasa de pelo. | Noh **oo**-seh **lah**-kah nee **grah**-sah deh **peh**-loh. |
| *You may eat normal* *meals.* | Puede comer su comida normal. | **Pweh**-deh koh-**mehr** soo koh-**mee**-dah nohr-**mahl**. |
| *I will apply disks* *on your scalp with a* *sticky paste.* | Le pondré discos de metal con una pasta en su cabeza. | Leh pohn-**dreh dees**-kohs deh meh-**tahl** kohn **oo**-nah **pahs**-tah ehn soo kah-**beh**-sah. |
| *I do not use needles;* *do not be afraid.* | No uso agujas; no tenga miedo. | Noh **oo**-soh ah-**goo**-hahs; noh **tehn**-gah **mee**-**eh**-doh. |
| *It is a simple test.* | Es un examen sencillo. | Ehs oon eg-**sah**-mehn sehn-**see**-yhoh. |
| *The EEG takes 1 to 2* *hours.* | El examen dura de 1 a 2 horas. | Ehl eg-**sag**-mehn **door**ah deh **oo**-nah ah dohs **oh**-rahs. |
| *Do not sleep for 24* *hours before the* *appointment.* | No duerma las 24 horas antes de la cita. | Noh **dwehr**-mah lahs vein-tee-**kwah**-troh **oh**rahs **ahn**-tehs deh lah **see**-tah. |
| *Please have someone* *come with you.* | Por favor traiga a alguien con usted. | Pohr fah-**vohr trah**-ee-gah ah ahl-**gee**-**ehn** kohn oos-**tehd**. |
| *You will need someone* *to drive you.* | Necesitará quien le maneje. | Neh-seh-see-tah-**rah** kee-ehn leh mah-**neh**-heh. |

Spinal Tap:

| | | |
|---|---|---|
| *I need to check your* *spinal fluid.* | Necesito ver como esta su líquido lumbar. | Neh-seh-**see**-toh vehr **koh**-moh **ehs**-tah soo **lee**-kee-doh loom-**bahr**. |
| *I need your written* *consent to do a spinal* *tap procedure.* | Necesito su firma de consentimiento para sacarle líquido de la columna. | Neh-seh-**see**-toh soo **feer**-mah deh kohn-sehn-tee-**mee**-**ehn**-toh **pah**-rah sah-**kahr**-leh **lee**-kee-doh deh lah koh-loom-nah. |
| *Please lie down on* *your side.* | Por favor acuéstese en su lado. | Pohr fah-**vohr** ah-**kwehs**-teh-seh ehn soo **lah**-doh. |
| *Bend your head* *forward.* | Doble la cabeza hacia al frente. | **Doh**-bleh lah kah-**beh**-sah ah-see-ah ehl **frehn**-teh. |
| *Pull up your knees to* *your stomach.* | Levante sus rodillas hacia su estómago. | Leh-**vahn**-teh soos roh-**dee**-yhahs **ah**-see-ah soo ehs-**toh**-mah-goh. |

| | | |
|---|---|---|
| I'm putting some medication to numb the area. | Voy a frotarle una medicina para entumecer el área. | Voy ah froh-**tahr**-leh **oo**-nah meh-dee-**see**-nah **pah**-rah ehn-too-meh-**sehr** ehl **ah**-reh-ah. |
| This should feel like a small needle stick. | Sentirá como un pequeño piquéte. | Sehn-tee-**rah koh**-moh oon peh-**keh**-nyoh pee-**keh**-teh. |
| Please tell me if any tingling or sensation occurs. | Por favor dígame si siente algún hormigeo o dolor. | Pohr fah-**vohr dee**-gah-meh see **see-ehn**-teh ahl-**goon** ohr-mee-**geh-oh** oh doh-**lohr**. |
| You need to stay in bed all day. | Necesita estar en cama todo el día. | Neh-seh-**see**-tah ehs-**tahr** ehn **kah**-mah **toh**-doh ehl **dee**-ah. |
| We are finished. | Acabamos. | Ah-kah-**bah**-mohs. |

Prescription Direction:

| | | |
|---|---|---|
| I'm going to prescribe some: | Voy a darle una receta para unas: | Voy ah **dahr**-leh **oo**-nah reh-**seh**-tah **pah**-rah **oo**-nahs: |
| * capsules. | * capsulas. | * **kap**-soo-lahs. |
| * pills. | * pildoras/pastillas. | * **peel**-doh-rahs/ pahs-**tee**-yhahs. |
| * suppositories. | * supositorios. | * **soo**-poh-see-**toh**-ree-ohs. |
| * tablets. | * tabletas. | * tah-**bleh**-tahs. |
| These are for your: | Estas son para su: | **Ehs**-tahs sohn **pah**-rah soo: |
| * illness | * enfermedad. | * ehn-**fehr**-meh-dad. |
| * infection. | * infección. | * een-feg-**see-ohn**. |
| * pain. | * dolor. | * doh-**lohr**. |
| Take ___ of these pills every ___ hours. | Tóme ___ de estas pastillas cada ___ horas. | **Toh**-meh ___ deh **ehs**-tahs pahs-**tee**-yhahs **kah**-dah ___ **oh**-rahs. |
| Take ___ of these pills every day. | Tóme ___ de estas pastillas todos los días. | **Toh**-meh ___ deh **ehs**-tahs pahs-**tee**-yhahs **toh**-dohs lohs **dee**-ahs. |
| Take ___ pill(s) daily for ___ days. | Tome ___ pastilla(s) diario por ___ días. | **Toh**-meh ___ pahs-**tee**-yhah(s) **dee-ah**-ree-oh pohr ___ **dee**-ahs. |

| English | Spanish | Pronunciation |
|---|---|---|
| You must take this medicine for ___ days. | Tiene que tomar esta medicina por ___ días. | Tee-eh-neh keh toh-mahr ehs-tah meh-dee-see-nah pohr ___ dee-ahs. |
| Take ___ to ___ tablets every ___ hours as needed. | Tóme de ___ a ___ tabletas cada ___ hora(s) como la necesite. | Toh-meh deh ___ ah ___ tah-bleh-tahs kah-dah oh-rah(s) koh-moh lah neh-seh-see-teh. |
| Use this anal or vaginal suppository every ___ hours. | Use este supositorio anal o vaginal cada ___ horas. | Oo-seh ehs-teh soo-poh-see-toh-ree-oh ah-nahl oh vah-hee-nahl kah-dah ___ oh-rahs. |
| Take ___ teaspoon every ___ hours for ___ days. | Tóme ___ cucharadita cada ___ horas por ___ días. | Toh-meh ___ koo-chah-rah-dee-tah kah-dah ___ oh-rahs pohr ___ dee-ahs. |
| Take ___ tablespoon every morning for ___ days. | Tóme ___ cucharada cada mañana por ___ días. | Toh-meh ___ koo-chah-rah-dah kah-dah mah-nyah-nah pohr ___ dee-ahs. |
| Take ___ Aspirin or ___ Tylenol for the pain or discomfort. | Tome ___ Aspirina o ___ Tilenol para el dolor de cabeza o malestar. | Toh-meh ___ Ahs-pee-ree-nah oh ___ Tee-leh-nohl pah-rah ehl doh-lohr deh kah-beh-sah oh mah-lehs-tahr. |

(See Appendix 1 for numbers)

| English | Spanish | Pronunciation |
|---|---|---|
| Here is some medication for diarrhea. | Estas son unas medicinas para la diarrea. | Ehs-tahs sohn oo-nahs meh-dee-see-nahs pah-rah lah dee-ah-rheh-ah. |
| Fill the dropper to this line and mix it with a glass of: | Llene éste gotero hasta la línea y mezclelo con: | Jeh-neh ehs-teh goh-teh-roh ahs-tah lah lee-neh-ah ee mehs-kleh-loh kohn: |
| * juice | * jugo | * hoo-goh |
| * milk | * leche | * leh-cheh |
| * water | * agua | * ah-gwah |
| Do not chew or crush the tablets. | No mastique o muela las tabletas. | Noh mahs-tee-keh oh mweh-lah lahs tah-bleh-tahs. |
| Do not take with: | No lo tome con: | Noh loh toh-meh kohn: |
| * antacids | * antiácidos | * ahn-tee-ah-see-dohs |
| * aspirin | * aspirina | * ahs-pee-ree-nah |
| * fruit juices | * jugos de frutas | * hoo-gohs deh froo-tahs |

| | | |
|---|---|---|
| * milk. | * leche | * **leh**-cheh |
| * orange juice | * jugo de naranja | * **hoo**-goh deh nah-**rahn**-hah |

## Prescription Information:

| | | |
|---|---|---|
| *Use these drops as directed.* | Use estas gotas como se las recetarón. | **Oo**-seh **ehs**-tahs **goh**-tahs **koh**-moh seh lahs reh-seh-**tah**-rohn. |
| *Keep refrigerated, but do not freeze.* | Mantenga refrigerado, pero no lo congele. | Mahn-**tehn**-gah reh-free-heh-**rah**-doh, **peh**-roh noh loh kohn-**heh**-leh. |
| *This may cause drowsiness.* | Esto puede causarle sueño. | **Ehs**-toh **pweh**-deh **kah**-oo-sahr-leh **sweh**-nyoh. |
| *Avoid alcohol with this medication.* | Evite el alcol con esta medicina. | Eh-**vee**-teh ehl ahl-**kohl** kohn **ehs**-tah meh-dee-**see**-nah. |
| *Exercise extreme caution when operating a machinery/automobile.* | Use precaución al manejar un automobil o maquinaria. | **Oo**-seh preh-kah-oo-**see**-**ohn** ahl mah-**neh**-hahr oon outoh-**moh**-beel oh mah-kee-**nah**-ree-ah. |
| *Drink more water while taking this medicine.* | Tóme mas agua mientras está con esta medicina. | **Toh**-meh mahs **ah**-gwah **mee**-**ehn**-trahs **ehs**-tah kohn **ehs**-tah meh-dee-**see**-nah. |
| *He has to drink plenty of fluids.* | El tiene que tomar mucho líquido. | Ehl **tee**-**eh**-neh keh toh-**mahr** **moo**-choh **lee**-kee-doh. |
| *Shake well before using.* | Agítelo bien antes de usar. | Ah-**hee**-teh-loh bee-ehn **ahn**-tehs deh oo-**sahr**. |
| *Take this medication 1/2 hour before/after meals.* | Tome esta medicina 1/2 hora antes/despues de comer. | **Toh**-meh **ehs**-tah meh-dee-**see**-nah **meh**-dee-ah **oh**-rah **ahn**-tehs/dehs-**pwehs** deh koh-**mehr**. |
| *Take before or after:* | Tóme ántes o despues: | **Toh**-meh **ahn**-tehs oh dehs-**pwehs**: |
| * bedtime | * de acostarse a dormir | * deh ah-kohs-**tahr**-seh ah dohr-**meer** |
| * breakfast | * del desayuno | * dehl **deh**-sah-you-noh |
| * dinner | * de la cena | * deh lah **seh**-nah |
| * lunch | * del almuerzo | * dehl ahl-**mwerh**-soh |

| | | |
|---|---|---|
| * meals. | * de las comidas | * deh lahs koh-**mee**-dahs |
| *Take this medication with food or milk.* | Tome esta medicina con leche o alimentos. | **Toh**-meh **ehs**-tah meh-dee-**see**-nah kohn **leh**-cheh oh ah-lee-**mehn**-tohs. |
| *Finish all the medication unless directed by your physician.* | Acábe toda la medicina a menos que su doctor le diga lo contrario. | Ah-**kah**-beh **toh**-dah lah meh-dee-**see**-nah ah **meh**-nohs keh soo **duck**-tohr leh **dee**gah loh kohn-**trah**-ree-oh. |
| *Keep out of reach of children.* | Manténgala lejos del alcance de los niños. | Mahn-**tehn**-gah-lah **leh**-hohs dehl ahl-**kahn**-seh deh lohs **nee**-nyohs. |
| *Limit your activities the next 24 hours.* | Limite sus actividades las próximas veinticuatro horas. | Lee-**mee**-teh soos ag-tee-vee-**dah**-dehs lahs **prog**-see-mahs **vein**-tee-**kwah**-troh **oh**-rahs. |

Emergency/Trauma Information:

| | | |
|---|---|---|
| *He is burned in over 80% of his body.* | Está quemado sobre ochenta por ciento del cuerpo. | Ehs-**tah** keh-**mah**-doh **soh**-breh oh-**chehn**-tah pohr **see-ehn**-toh dehl **kwehr**-poh. |
| *He has burns of:* | El tiene quemadas de: | Ehl **tee-eh**-neh keh-**mah**-dahs deh: |
| * first degree | * primer grado | * pree-**mehr grah**-doh |
| * second degree | * segundo grado | * seh-**goon**-doh **grah**-doh |
| * third degree | * tercer grado | * tehr-**sehr grah**-doh |
| *He/She is bleeding from:* | El/Ella está sangrando en: | Ehl/Eh-yhah ehs-**tah** sahn-**grahn**-doh ehn: |
| * head | * la cabeza | * lah kah-**beh**-sah |
| * stomach | * el estómago | * ehl ehs-**toh**-mah-goh |
| * internally | * internamente | * een-**tehr**-nah-mehn-teh |
| * a bullet wound | * de una herida de bala | * deh **oo**-nah eh-**ree**-dah deh **bah**-lah |
| *He/She has a:* | El/Ella tiene una: | Ehl/Eh-yhah **tee-eh**-neh **oo**-nah: |
| * laceration | * laceracion | * lah-seh-rah-**see-ohn** |
| * gash | * cuchillada | * koo-chee-**yhah**-dah |

| | | |
|---|---|---|
| * puncture wound | * herida perforada | * eh-**ree**-dah pehr-foh-**rah**-dah |
| *He/She will need a* blood transfusion. | El/Ella necesita una transfusion de sangre. | Ehl/Eh-yhah neh-seh-**see**-tah **oo**-nah trans-foo-**see**-**ohn** deh **sahn**-greh. |
| *What is his/her* blood type? | Cuál es su tipo de sangre? | **Kwahl** ehs soo **tee**-poh deh **sahn**-greh? |
| *We need to operate* immediately to: | Necesitamos operar de inmediato para: | Neh-seh-see-**tah**-mohs oh-peh-**rahr** deh een-meh-**dee**-**ah**-toh **pah**-rah: |
| * stop the bleeding | * parar la sangre | * pah-**rahr** lah **sahn**-greh |
| * take out the bullet | * sacar la bala | * sah-**kahr** lah **bah**-lah |
| *Do you understand me?* | Me entiende? | Meh ehn-**tee**-**ehn**-deh? |
| *The wound (cut) needs* stitches. | La herida (cortadura) necesita puntadas. | Lah eh-**ree**-dah (kohr-tah-**doo**-rah) neh-seh-**see**-tah poon-**tah**-dahs. |
| *Keep the wound* area dry | Mantenga la herida y area seca. | Mahn-**tehn**-gah lah eh-**ree**-dah ee **ah**-reh-ah **seh**-kah. |
| *Do not get the wound* wet. | No se moje la herida. | Noh seh **moh**-heh lah eh-**ree**-dah. |

*Cardinal Numbers*

| | | |
|---|---|---|
| Zero | Cero | **Seh**-roh |
| One | Uno | **Oo**-noh |
| Two | Dos | Dohs |
| Three | Tres | Trehs |
| Four | Cuatro | **Kwah**-troh |
| Five | Cinco | **Seen**-koh |
| Six | Seis | Says |
| Seven | Siete | **See-eh**-teh |
| Eight | Ocho | **Oh**-choh |
| Nine | Nueve | **Nweh**-veh |
| Ten | Diez | Dee-ehs |
| Eleven | Once | **Ohn**-seh |
| Twelve | Doce | **Doh**-seh |
| Thirteen | Trece | **Treh**-seh |
| Fourteen | Catorce | Kah-**tohr**-seh |
| Fifteen | Quince | **Keen**-seh |
| Sixteen | Dieciseis | **Dee-eh**-see-says |
| Seventeen | Diecisiete | **Dee-eh**-see-**see-eh**-teh |
| Eighteen | Dieciocho | **Dee-eh**-see-**oh**-choh |
| Nineteen | Diecinueve | **Dee-eh**-see-**nweh**-veh |
| Twenty | Veinte | **Vein**-teh |
| Twenty one | Veintiuno | **Vein**-tee-**oo**-noh |
| Twenty two | Veintidos | **Vein**-tee-dohs |
| Thirty | Treinta | **Treh-een**-tah |
| Forty | Cuarenta | Kwah-**rehn**-tah |
| Fifty | Cinquenta | Seen-**kwehn**-tah |
| Sixty | Sesenta | Seh-**sehn**-tah |
| Seventy | Setenta | Seh-**tehn**-tah |
| Eighty | Ochenta | Oh-**chehn**-tah |
| Ninety | Noventa | Noh-**vehn**-tah |
| One Hundred | Cien | See-**ehn** |

| | | |
|---|---|---|
| What time is it? | Que hora es? | Keh **oh**-rah ehs? |
| It is 1:13 p.m. | Es la una y trece de la tarde. | Ehs lah **oo**-nah ee **treh**-seh deh lah **tahr**-deh. |

## *Ordinal Numbers*

| | | |
|---|---|---|
| First | Primero | Pree-**meh**-roh |
| Second | Segundo | Seh-**goon**-doh |
| Third | Tercero | Tehr-**seh**-roh |
| Fourth | Cuarto | **Kwahr**-toh |
| Fifth | Quinto | **Keen**-toh |
| Sixth | Sexto | **Seg**-toh |
| Septimo | Sextimo | **Seg**-tee-moh |
| Eighth | Octavo | **Og**-tah-voh |
| Ninth | Noveno | Noh-**veh**-noh |
| Tenth | Decimo | **Deh**-see-moh |
| Eleventh | Undecimo | Oon-**deh**-see-moh |
| Twelfth | Duodecimo | Dwoh-**deh**-see-moh |
| Thirteenth | Decimo tercero | **Deh**-see-moh tehr-**seh**-roh |
| Fourteenth | Decimo cuarto | **Deh**-see-moh **kwahr**-toh |
| Twentieth | Vigesimo | Vee-**heh**-see-moh |
| Twenty-first | Vigesimo primero | Vee-**heh**-see-moh pree-**meh**-roh |

*Days of the Week*

| | | |
|---|---|---|
| Sunday | Domingo | Doh-**meen**-goh |
| Monday | Lunes | **Loo**-nehs |
| Tuesday | Martes | **Mahr**-tehs |
| Wednesday | Miércoles | **Mee-ehr**-koh-lehs |
| Thursday | Jueves | **Hweh**-vehs |
| Friday | Viernes | **Vee-ehr**-nehs |
| Saturday | Sabado | **Sah**-bah-doh |
| What day is today? | Que dia es hoy? | Keh **dee**-ah ehs oy (as in joy but without the j)? |
| Today is.... | Hoy es.... | Oy ehs.... |

*Months of the Year*

| | | |
|---|---|---|
| January | Enero | Eh-**neh**-roh |
| February | Febrero | Feh-**breh**-roh |
| March | Marzo | **Mahr**-soh |
| April | Abril | Ah-**breel** |
| May | Mayo | **Mah**-yoh |
| June | Junio | **Hoo**-nee-oh |
| July | Julio | **Hoo**-lee-oh |
| August | Agosto | Ah-**gohs**-toh |
| September | Septiembre | Sep-**tee-ehm**-breh |
| October | Octubre | Og-**too**-breh |
| November | Noviembre | Noh-**vee-ehm**-breh |
| December | Diciembre | Dee-**see-ehm**-breh |
| What month are we on? | En que mes estamos? | Ehn keh mehs ehs-**tah**-mohs? |
| The month is | El mes es.... | Ehl mehs ehs.... |

82

*Guide to Certain Letters of the Alphabet and their Pronunciation*

Spanish is a language pronounced generally just as it is written. Few exceptions are noted, however. They are:

"C"     Pronounce it hard before the consonants "a", "o" and "u": cama (**kah**-mah), costa (**kohs**-tah), cuesta (**kwehs**-tah). Pronunce it soft before the consonants "e" and "i": dulce (**dool**-seh), cien (see-ehn).

"G"     The same rule as in "C" applies to the letter "G". Pronounce it hard before the consonants "a", "o" and "u": gas, goma (**goh**-mah), gusto (**goos**-toh). Pronounce it soft (as in the 'H' in English) before the consonants "e" and "i": gema (**heh**-mah), gimnasia (him-**nah**-see-ah).

"H"     Pay no attention to this letter as it is silent.

"J"     Follows the 'H' sound of English.

"Ll"    You will find double "ll" in words as in lluvia (**you**-vee-ah) and llave (**yhah**-veh). It is a nasal sound pronounced like the 'Y' (you) in English.

"Ñ"     Is a nasal sound similar to the 'Y' in English preceded by the letter N as in caNYon. You will find it in the word mañana (mah-**nyah**-nah). For example, "I'll be seein' ya".

"RR"    Pronounce it with a hard roll of your tongue.

"V"     In some countries, it is pronounce the same as the letter 'B'.

"Z"     Pronounce the same way as the letter 'S'.

One must always be careful when pronouncing a word, since a word, if pronounced slightly different, can have two meanings whereby creating embarrassing moments. For instance, the words pelo (**peh**-low ‹hair›) and pedo (**peh**-doh ‹flatus›); ano (**ah**-noh ‹anus›) and año (**ah**-nyòh ‹year›); pero (**peh**-roh ‹but›) and perro (**peh**-rhoh ‹dog›).

Nouns in Spanish are generally viewed as male or female. If the word ends with the letter "o", it is considered to be male; if the word ends with the letter "a" it is considered female.

| English | Spanish | Pronunciation |
|---|---|---|
| Acquired Immuno Deficiency Syndrome - (AIDS) | Síndrome Immuno-lógico de Deficiencias Adquirida (SIDA) | **Seen**-droh-meh Een-moo-noh-**loh**-hee-koh deh Deh-fee-**see-ehn**-see-ahs Ad-kee-**ree**-dahs (**See**-dah) |
| abdomen | abdomen | ab-**doh**-mehn |
| abortion | aborto | ah-**bohr**-toh |
| abuse | abuso | ah-**boo**-soh |
| accident | accidente | ag-see-**dehn**-teh |
| all | todo | **toh**-doh |
| allergy | alérgia | ah-**lehr**-hee-ah |
| always | siempre | **see-ehm**-preh |
| amygdala | amígdala | ah-**meeg**-dah-lah |
| (toncils are also called amygdalas in Spanish) | | |
| and | y | ee |
| anesthesiologist | anestesiólogo | ah-**nehs**-teh-**see-oh**-loh-goh |
| anesthetist | anestesista | ah-**nehs**-teh-**sees**-tah |
| ankle(s) | tobillo(s) | toh-**bee**-yhoh(s) |
| anus | ano | ah-noh |
| anxiety | ansiedad | ahn-**see-eh**-dad |
| any | alguno | ahl-**goo**-noh |
| appendicitis | apendicitis | ah-**pehn**-dee-**see**-tees |
| appendix | apéndice | ah-**pehn**-dee-seh |
| arm | brazo | **brah**-soh |
| arrhythmia | aritmia cardíaca | ah-**reet**-mee-ah hahr-**dee-ah**-kah |
| artery(ies) | arteria(s) | ahr-**teh**-ree-ah(s) |
| asphyxia | asfixia | ahs-**feeg**-see-ah |
| asthma | asma | **ahs**-mah |
| at | en; a | ehn; ah |
| back | espalda | ehs-**pahl**-dah |
| bad | malo | **mah**-loh |
| because | porque | pohr-**keh** |
| before | antes | **ahn**-tehs |
| better | mejor | meh-**hohr** |
| bile | bilis | **bee**-lees |
| bladder | vejiga | veh-**hee**-gah |
| blister | ampolla | ahm-**poh**-yah |
| blood | sangre | **sahn**-greh |
| body | cuerpo | **kwehr**-poh |
| bone(s) | hueso(s) | **weh**-soh(s) |
| bowels | fece(s)/ evacuaciones | **feh**-seh(s) eh-vah-kwah-**see-oh**-nehs |
| brain | cerebro | seh-**reh**-broh |
| breast | busto/seno | **boos**-toh/**seh**-noh |
| breath | aliento | ah-lee-**ehn**-toh |
| breathe | respirar | rehs-pee-**rahr** |
| bronchitis | bronquitis | brohn-**kee**-tees |
| bruise | magulla | mah-**goo**-yhah |
| bump | chichón/chichote | chee-**chohn**/chee-**choh**-teh |
| burn(s) | quemada(s) | keh-**mah**-dah(s) |
| but | pero | **peh**-roh |
| buttocks | nalgas | **nahl**-gahs |
| cancer | cancer | **kahn**-sehr |

| | | |
|---|---|---|
| cardiologist | cardiólogo | kahr-**dee-oh**-loh-goh |
| cheek | mejilla | meh-**hee**-yhah |
| chest | pecho | **peh**-choh |
| chicken pox | varicela (la china) | vah-ree-**seh**-lah (lah **chee**-nah) |
| chills | escalofrios | ehs-kah-loh-**free-ohs** |
| chin | barbilla | bahr-**bee**-yhah |
| cold | catarro/frio | kah-**tah**-rhoh/**free**-oh |
| constipation | estreñimiento | ehs-treh-nyee-**mee-ehn**-toh |
| constipation | constipación | kohns-tee-pah-**see-ohn** |
| convulsions | convulsiones | kohn-vool-**see-oh**-nehs |
| cough | toser/tos | toh-**sehr**/tohs |
| cramp | calambre | kah-**lahm**-breh |
| cyst | quiste | **kees**-teh |
| dentist | dentista | dehn-**tees**-tah |
| dermatologist | dermatólogo | dehr-mah-**toh**-loh-goh |
| diabetes | diabetes | dee-ah-**beh**-tehs |
| diarrhea | diarrea | dee-ah-**rhe-ah** |
| discharge | secresión | seh-kreh-**see-ohn** |
| discomfort | malestar | mah-lehs-**tahr** |
| dizziness | maréos | mah-**reh**-ohs |
| dizzy | mareo | mah-**reh**-oh |
| drug | droga | **droh**-gah |
| drug addiction | narcomania | nahr-koh-mah-**nee-ah** |
| during | durante | doo-**rahn**-teh |
| earache | dolor de oído | doh-**lohr** deh oh-**ee**-doh |
| early | temprano | tehm-**prah**-noh |
| elbow | codo | **koh**-doh |
| endocrinologist | endocrinólogo | ehn-doh-kree-**noh**-loh-goh |
| epilepsy | epilepsia | ehpee-**lep**-see-ah |
| esophagus | esófago | eh-**soh**-fah-goh |
| examine | examinar | eg-sah-**mee**-nahr |
| excuse me | con permiso | kohn pehr-**mee**-soh |
| extremity(ies) | extremidad(es) | egs-**treh**-mee-dad(ehs) |
| eye(s) | ojo(s) | **oh**-hoh(s) |
| face | cara | **kah**-rah |
| faint | desmayo | dehs-**mah**-yhoh |
| fainting spell | desvanecimiento | **dehs**-vah-neh-see-mee-**ehn**-toh |
| family practitioner | médico de familia | **meh**-dee-koh deh fah-**mee**-lee-ah |
| far | lejos | **leh**-hohs |
| feet | pies | pee-ehs |
| fever | fiebre/calentura | **fee-eh**-breh/kah-lehn-**too**-rah |
| finger | dedo | **deh**-doh |
| foot | pié | pee-eh |
| for | para; por | **pah**-rah; pohr |
| forehead | frente | **frehn**-teh |
| forgive me | perdóneme | pehr-**doh**-neh-meh |
| fracture | fractura | frag-**too**-rah |
| from | de; desde | deh; **dehs**-deh |
| gall bladder | vesícula | veh-**see**-koo-lah |
| gash | cuchillada | koo-chee-**yhah**-dah |
| general practitioner | médico general | **meh**-dee-koh heh-neh-rahl |
| german measles | rubeola | roo-**beh-oh**-lah |
| gonorrhea | gonorrea | goh-noh-**rheh-ah** |
| good | bueno | **bweh**-noh |
| gout | gota | **goh**-tah |

| gynecologist | ginecólogo | hee-neh-**koh**-loh-goh |
| hand(s) | mano(s) | **mah**-noh(s) |
| head | cabeza | kah-**beh**-sah |
| headache | dolor de cabeza | doh-**lohr** deh kah-**beh**-sah |
| heart | corazón | koh-rah-**sohn** |
| heart attack | ataque al corazón | ah-**tah**-keh ahl koh-rah-**sohn** |
| heartburn | acidez estomacal | ah-see-**dehs** ehs-toh-mah-**kahl** |
| heel | talón | tah-**lohn** |
| hematologist | hematólogo | heh-mah-**toh**-loh-goh |
| hemorrhage | hemorragia | eh-moh-**rrah**-hee-ah |
| hemorrhoids | almorranas | ahl-moh-**rrah**-nahs |
| | (hemorroides) | (eh-moh-**roy**-dehs) |
| high blood pressure | presión alta | preh-**see**—ohn **ahl**-tah |
| hip(s) | cadera(s) | kah-**deh**—rah(s) |
| hives | urticarias | oohr-tee-**kah**-ree-ahs |
| hoarseness | ronquera | rohn-**keh**-rah |
| how | como | **koh**-moh |
| hurt | daño | dah-**nyoh** |
| hypertension | hipertensión | ee-pehr-tehn-**see**-**ohn** |
| I don't understand | no entiendo | noh ehn-**tee**—**ehn**-doh |
| if/yes | si | see |
| in | en | ehn |
| indigestion | indigestion | **een**-dee-hehs-**tee**-**ohn** |
| infarct | infarto | een-**fahr**-toh |
| infection | infección | een-feg-**see**-**ohn** |
| inflammation | inflamación | een-flah-mah-**see**-**ohn** |
| injection | inyección | een-**jeg**-**see**-**ohn** |
| injury | herida/daño | eh-**ree**-dah/**dah**-nyoh |
| insomnio | insomnia | een-**some**-nee-ah |
| internist | internista | een-tehr-**nees**-tah |
| intestin(es) | intestino(s) | een-tehs-tee-noh(s) |
| jaw | quijada | kee-**hah**-dah |
| joint | coyuntura/nudo | koh-yoon-**too**-rah/**noo**-doh |
| kidney(s) | riñon(es) | ree-**nyohn**(ehs) |
| knee(s) | rodilla(s) | roh-**dee**-yhah(s) |
| laryngitis | laringitis | lah-reehn-**hee**-tees |
| late | tarde | **tahr**-deh |
| lately | ultimamente | **ool**-tee-mah-**mehn**-teh |
| leg(s) | pierna(s) | **pee**-**ehr**-nah(s) |
| less | menos | **meh**-nohs |
| listen | oye | **oh**-yheh |
| little | poco | **poh**-koh |
| liver | higado | **ee**-gah-doh |
| low blood pressure | presión baja | preh-**see**-**ohn** **bah**-hah |
| lung(s) | pulmón(es) | pool-**mohn**(ehs) |
| mandible | mandibula | mahn-**dee**-boo-lah |
| measles | sarampión | sah-rahm-**pee**-**ohn** |
| medicine | medicina | meh-dee-**see**-nah |
| miscarriage | malparto | mahl-**pahr**-toh |
| mouth | boca | **boh**-kah |
| much/many | mucho | **moo**-choh |
| mumps | paperas | pah-**peh**-rahs |
| muscle(s) | músculo(s) | **moos**-koo-loh(s) |
| nail(s) | uña(s) | **oo**-nyah(s) |
| nasal Drip | goteo nasal | goh-**teh**-oh nah-**sahl** |

| English | Spanish | Pronunciation |
|---------|---------|---------------|
| nausea | nauseas/basca | nah-oo-seh-ahs/**bahs**-kah |
| navel | ombligo | ohm-**blee**-goh |
| near | cerca | **sehr**-kah |
| neck | cuello | **kweh**-yoh |
| nervousness | nerviosismo | nehr-vee-oh-**sees**-moh |
| neurologist | neurólogo | neh-oo-**roh**-loh-goh |
| never | nunca | **noon**-kah |
| nipple | pezón | peh-**sohn** |
| nose | nariz | nah-**rees** |
| not so fast | no tan rapido | noh tahn **rah**-pee-doh |
| nothing | nada | **nah**-dah |
| now | ahora | ah-**oh**-rah |
| obstetritian | obstétrico | obs-**teh**-tree-koh |
| of | de | deh |
| often | frecuente | freh-**kwehn**-teh |
| okay | de acuerdo | deh ah-**kwehr**-doh |
| oncologist | oncólogo | ohn-**koh**-loh-goh |
| operation | operación | oh-peh-rah-**see-ohn** |
| ophthalmologist | oftalmólogo | of-tahl-**moh**-log-goh |
| optometrist | optometrista | op-toh-meh-**treehs**-tah |
| or | o | oh |
| orthodontist | ortodoncista | ohr-toh-dohn-**sees**-tah |
| orthopedist | ortopedista | ohr-toh-peh-**dees**-tah |
| otolaryngologist | otorrinolaringólogo | oh-toh-**rhee**-noh-lahn-reen-**goh**-loh-goh |
| pain | dolor | doh-**lohr** |
| paralysis | parálisis | pah-**rah**-lee-sees |
| pathologist | patólogo | pah-**toh**-loh-goh |
| pediatrist | pediátrico | peh-**dee-ah**-tree-koh |
| pharmacist | farmacéutico | fahr-mah-**seh-oo**-tee-koh |
| pharmacologist | farmacólogo | fahr-mah-**koh**-loh-goh |
| pill | pastilla/pildora | pahs-**tee**-yah/peel-**doh**-rah |
| plastic surgeon | cirujano plástico | see-roo-**hah**-noh **plahs**-tee-koh |
| please | por favor | pohr fah-**vohr** |
| podiatrist | podiátrico | poh-**dee-ah**-tree-koh |
| poison | veneno | veh-**neh**-noh |
| pregnant | embarazada | ehm-**bah**-rah-**sah**-dah |
| psychiatrist | psiquiátrico | see-**kee-ah**-tree-koh |
| psychologist | psicólogo | see-**koh**-loh-goh |
| pulse | pulso | **pool**-soh |
| radiologist | radiólogo | rah-**dee-oh**-loh-goh |
| rare | raro | **rah**-roh |
| rash | salpullido | sahl-poo-**yee**-doh |
| rectum | recto | **reg**-toh |
| relax | relaje | reh-**lah**-heh |
| sample | especimen | ehs-**peh**-see-mehn |
| scalp | cabellera | kah-beh-**yheh**-rah |
| seizure(s) | convulsion(es) | **kohn**-vool-**see-ohn**-(ehs) |
| shakiness | temblores | tehm-**bloh**-rehs |
| shoulder | hombro | **ohm**-broh |
| since | desde | **dehs**-deh |
| sinusitis | sinusitis | see-noo-**see**-tees |
| skeleton | esqueleto | ehs-**keh**-leh-toh |
| skin | piel | pee-ehl |
| skull | cráneo | **krah**-neh-oh |

| sleep | dormir | dohr-**meer** |
| slow | despacio | Dehs-**pah**-see-oh |
| smallpox | viruela | vee-**rweh**-lah |
| sneeze | estornudar | ehs-tohr-noo-**dahr** |
| sometime | alguna vez | ahl-**goo**-nah vehs |
| soon | pronto | **prohn**-toh |
| sore | llaga | **yah**-gah |
| sore throat | dolor de garganta | doh-**lohr** deh gahr-**gahn**-tah |
| sorry | lo siento | loh **see-ehn**-toh |
| specimen | muestra/espécimen | **mwehs**-trah/ehs-**peh**-see-mehn |
| spine | columna vertebral/ espinazo | koh-**loom**-nah vehr-**teh**-brahl/ ehs-**pee**-nah-soh |
| spit | escupir/saliva | ehs-koo-**peer**/sah-**lee**-vah |
| spleen | bazo | **bah**-soh |
| sprain | torcer | tohr-**sehr** |
| sputum | esputos | ehs-**poo**-tohs |
| stiff | rígido | **ree**-hee-doh |
| stitch | puntada/puntos | poon-**tah**-dah/**poon**-tohs |
| stomach | estómago | ehs-**toh**-mah-goh |
| stomach ache | dolor de estómago | doh-**lohr** deh ehs-**toh**-mah-goh |
| stool | excremento/caca | egs-kreh-**mehn**-toh/**kah**-kah |
| stress | tensión | tehn-**see-ohn** |
| stroke | ataque/derrame | ah-**tah**-keh/deh-rhah-meh |
| suicide | suicidio | swee-**see**-dee-oh |
| surgeon | cirujano | see-roo-**hah**-noh |
| surgery | operación | oh-peh-rah-**see-ohn** |
| swallow | tragar | trah-**gahr** |
| sweat | sudor | soo-**dohr** |
| swelling | hinchazón | een-chah-**sohn** |
| syphilis | sífilis | **see**-fee-lees |
| tachycardia | taquicardia | **tah**-kee-**kahr**-dee-ah |
| temple | sien | see-ehn |
| than | que | keh |
| thank you | gracias | **grah**-see-ahs |
| the | el (sigular masculine) | ehl |
| | la (singular femine) | lah |
| | las (plural feminine) | lahs |
| | los (plural masculine) | lohs |
| therapist | terapista | teh-rah-**pees**-tah |
| thigh | muslo | **moos**-loh |
| throat | garganta | gahr-**gahn**-tah |
| thyroid | tiroide | tee-**roy**-deh |
| tingle | hormigueo | ohr-mee-**geh**-oh |
| tired | cansado | kahn-**sah**-doh |
| to | a | ah |
| today | hoy | oy |
| toe | dedo del pie | **deh**-doh dehl pee-**eh** |
| toes | dedos de los pies | **deh**-dohs deh lohs pee-ehs |
| tomorrow | mañana | mah-**nyah**-nah |
| tongue | lengua | **lehn**-gwah |

| | | |
|---|---|---|
| tonsillitis | tonsilitis/anginas | tohn-see-**lee**-tees/ahn-**hee**-nahs |
| tonsils | anginas | ahn-**hee**-nahs |
| tooth ache | dolor de muela | doh-**lohr** deh **mweh**-lah |
| trachea | tráquea | **trah**-keh-ah |
| transfusion | transfusión | trahns-foo-**see-ohn** |
| tremors | temblores | tehm-**bloh**-rehs |
| trunk | tronco | **trohn**-koh |
| ulcer(s) | úlcera(s) | ool-**seh**-rah(s) |
| unconcious | inconciente | een-kohn-**see-ehn**-teh |
| ureter | uréter | oo-**reh**-tehr |
| urethra | uretra | oo-**reh**trah |
| urine | orina | oh-**ree**-nah |
| urologist | urólogo | oo-**roh**-loh-goh |
| uterus | útero | **oo**-teh-roh |
| vagina | vagina | vah-**hee**-nah |
| vein(s) | vena(s) | veh-**nah(s)** |
| venereal disease | enfermedad venérea | **ehn**-fehr-meh-**dad** |
| | | veh-**neh**-reh-ah |
| very | muy | mooy |
| waist | cintura | seen-**too**-rah |
| weak | debil | **deh**-beel |
| weakness | debilidad | deh-bee-lee-**dad** |
| weight | peso | **peh**-soh |
| well | bien | bee-ehn |
| what | que | keh |
| wheezy | silbido de asma | seel-**bee**-doh deh **ahs**-mah |
| which | cual | kwahl |
| whooping cough | tos ferina | tohs feh-**ree**-nah |
| why | porque | pohr-**keh** |
| without | sin | seen |
| womb | matriz | mah-**trees** |
| worse/worst | peor | peh-**ohr** |
| wound | herida | eh-**ree**-dah |
| wrist | muñeca | moo-**nyeh**-kah |
| yesterday | ayer | ah-**yhehr** |

| | | |
|---|---|---|
| abdomen | ab-**doh**-mehn | abdomen |
| aborto | ah-**bohr**-toh | abortion |
| abuso | ah-**boo**-soh | abuse |
| accidente | ag-see-**dehn**-teh | accident |
| alérgia | ah-**lehr**-hee-ah | allergy |
| aliento | ah-lee-**ehn**-toh | breath |
| anginas | ahn-**hee**-nahs | toncils |
| ano | ah-noh | anus |
| ansiedad | ahn-**see-eh**-dad | anxiety |
| apéndice | ah-**pehn**-dee-seh | appendix |
| arteria(s) | ahr-**teh**-ree-ah(s) | artery(ies) |
| ataque/derrame | ah-**tah**-keh/deh-rhah-meh | stroke |
| barbilla | bahr-**bee**-yhah | chin |
| bazo | **bah**-soh | spleen |
| bilis | **bee**-lees | bile |
| boca | **boh**-kah | mouth |
| brazo | **brah**-soh | arm |
| busto/seno | **boos**-toh/**seh**-noh | breast |
| cabellera | kah-beh-**yheh**-rah | scalp |
| cabeza | kah-**beh**-sah | head |
| cadera(s) | kah-**deh**-rah(s) | hip(s) |
| cansado | kahn-**sah**-doh | tired |
| cara | **kah**-rah | face |
| catarro/frio | kah-**tah**-rhoh/**free**-oh | cold |
| cerebro | seh-**reh**-broh | brain |
| cintura | seen-**too**-rah | waist |
| codo | **koh**-doh | elbow |
| columna vertebral | koh-**loom**-nah vehr-**teh**-brahl | spine |
| convulsion(es) | kohn-vool-**see-ohn**-(ehs) | seizure(s) |
| corazón | koh-rah-**sohn** | heart |
| coyuntura/nudo | koh-yoon-**too**-rah/**noo**-doh | joint |
| cráneo | **krah**-neh-oh | skull |
| cuchillada | koo-chee-**yhah**-dah | gash |
| cuello | **kweh**-yoh | neck |
| cuerpo | **kwehr**-poh | body |
| daño | dah-**nyoh** | hurt |
| debil | **deh**-beel | weak |
| debilidad | deh-bee-lee-**dad** | weakness |
| dedo | **deh**-doh | finger |
| dedos de los pies | **deh**-dohs deh lohs pee-ehs | toes |
| desmayo | dehs-**mah**-yhoh | faint |
| desvanecimiento | **dehs**-vah-neh-see-mee-**ehn**-toh | fainting spell |
| dolor | doh-**lohr** | pain |
| dolor de oido | doh-**lohr** deh oh-**ee**-do | earache |
| dormir | dohr-**meer** | sleep |
| droga | **droh**-gah | drug |
| embarazada | ehm-**bah**-rah-**sah**-dah | pregnant |
| escalofrios | ehs-kah-loh-**free**-ohs | chills |
| escupir/saliva | ehs-koo-**peer**/sah-**lee**-vah | spit |
| esófago | eh-**soh**-fah-goh | esophagus |
| espalda | ehs-**pahl**-dah | back |
| especimen | ehs-**peh**-see-mehn | sample |

| | | |
|---|---|---|
| espinazo | ehs-**pee**-nah-soh | spine |
| esputos | ehs-**poo**-tohs | sputum |
| esqueleto | ehs-**keh**-leh-toh | skeleton |
| estornudar | ehs-tohr-noo-**dahr** | sneeze |
| estómago | ehs-**toh**-mah-goh | stomach |
| estreñimiento | ehs-treh-nyee-**mee**-ehn-toh | constipation |
| examinar | eg-sah-**mee**-nahr | examine |
| excremento/caca | egs-kreh-**mehn**-toh/**kah**-kah | stool |
| extremidad(es) | egs-**treh**-mee-dah(dehs) | extremity(ies) |
| feces/ | **feh**-sehs/ | bowels |
| evacuaciones | eh-vah-kwah-**see**-**oh**-nehs | |
| fiebre | **fee**-**eh**-breh | fever |
| fractura | frag-**too**-rah | fracture |
| frente | **frehn**-teh | forehead |
| garganta | gahr-**gahn**-tah | throat |
| herida | eh-**ree**-dah | wound |
| herida/daño | eh-**ree**-dah/**dah**-nyoh | injury |
| hinchazón | een-chah-**sohn** | swelling |
| hígado | **ee**-gah-doh | liver |
| hombro | **ohm**-broh | shoulder |
| hormigueo | ohr-mee-**geh**-oh | tingle |
| hueso(s) | **weh**-soh(s) | bone(s) |
| inconciente | een-kohn-**see**-**ehn**-teh | unconscious |
| indigestion | **een**-dee-hehs-**tee**-**ohn** | indigestion |
| intestinos | **een**-tehs-**tee**-nohs | intestines |
| inyección | een-**jeg**-**see**-**ohn** | injection |
| lengua | **lehn**-gwah | tongue |
| llaga | **yah**-gah | sore |
| magulla | mah-**goo**-yhah | bruise |
| malparto | mahl-**pahr**-toh | miscarriage |
| mandibula | mahn-**dee**-boo-lah | mandible |
| mano(s) | **mah**-noh(s) | hand(s) |
| mareo | mah-**reh**-oh | dizzy |
| matriz | mah-**trees** | womb |
| medicina | meh-dee-**see**-nah | medicine |
| mejilla | meh-**hee**-yhah | cheek |
| muestra/espécimen | **mwehs**-trah/ehs-**peh**-see-mehn | specimen |
| muñeca | moo-**nyeh**-kah | wrist |
| muslo | **moos**-loh | thigh |
| músculo(s) | **moos**-koo-loh(s) | muscle(s) |
| nalgas | **nahl**-gahs | buttocks |
| nariz | nah-**rees** | nose |
| nausea | nah-**oo**-seah | nausea |
| ojos | **oh**-hohs | eyes |
| ombligo | ohm-**blee**-goh | navel |
| operación | oh-peh-rah-**see**-**ohn** | operation/surgery |
| orina | oh-**ree**-nah | urine |
| pastilla/pildora | pahs-**tee**-yah/peel-**doh**-rah | pill |
| pecho | **peh**-choh | chest |
| peso | **peh**-soh | weight |
| pezón | peh-**sohn** | nipple |
| piel | pee-**ehl** | skin |
| pierna(s) | pee-**ehr**-nah(s) | leg(s) |
| pies | pee-ehs | feet |
| pié | pee-eh | foot |

| Spanish | Pronunciation | English |
|---|---|---|
| presión alta | preh-**see-ohn ahl**-tah | high blood pressure |
| presión baja | preh-**see-ohn bah**-hah | low blood pressure |
| pulmón(es) | pool-**mohn**(ehs) | lung(s) |
| pulso | **pool**-soh | pulse |
| puntada/puntos | poon-**tah**-dah/**poon**-tohs | stitch |
| quemada(s) | keh-**mah**-dah(s) | burn(s) |
| quijada | kee-**hah**-dah | jaw |
| recto | **reg**-toh | rectum |
| relaje | reh-**lah**-heh | relax |
| respirar | rehs-pee-**rahr** | breathe |
| riñon(es) | ree-**nyohn**(ehs) | kidney(s) |
| rígido | **ree**-hee-doh | stiff |
| rodilla(s) | roh-**dee**-yhah(s) | knee(s) |
| sangre | **sahn**-greh | blood |
| secresión | seh-kreh-**see-ohn** | discharge |
| sien | see-ehn | temple |
| silbido de asma | seel-**bee**-doh deh **ahs**-mah | wheezy |
| sudor | soo-**dohr** | sweat |
| suicidio | swee-**see**-dee-oh | suicide |
| talón | tah-**lohn** | heel |
| temblores | tehm-**bloh**-rehs | shakiness/tremors |
| tensión | tehn-**see-ohn** | tension |
| tiroide | tee-**roy**-deh | thyroid |
| tobillo(s) | toh-**bee**-yhoh(s) | ankle(s) |
| torcer | tohr-**sehr** | sprain |
| tragar | trah-**gahr** | swallow |
| transfusión | trahns-foo-**see-ohn** | transfusion |
| tráquea | **trah**-keh-ah | trachea |
| tronco | **trohn**-koh | trunk |
| uña(s) | **oo**-nyah(s) | nail(s) |
| uretra | oo-**reh**-trah | urethra |
| uréter | oo-**reh**-tehr | ureter |
| urticarias | oohr-tee-**kah**-ree-ahs | hives |
| útero | **oo**-teh-roh | uterus |
| vagina | vah-**hee**-nah | vagina |
| vejiga | veh-**hee**-gah | bladder |
| vena(s) | **veh**-nah(s) | vein(s) |
| veneno | veh-**neh**-noh | poison |
| vesícula | veh-**see**-koo-lah | gall bladder |

INDEX OF SIGNS AND SYMPTOMS

Abdominal
    pain, 45, 47
    distention, 45
    swelling, 48
Abortion, history of, 54
Ache
    stomach, 46
    joint, 51
Aching pain, 5, 28, 37
Agitation, 56
AIDS, 12
Alcohol,
    abuse, 12, 13
    use, 65
Allergens, exposure to, 9
Allergy to
    penicillin, 11, 52
    bee or hornet stings, 11
Allergy, history of, 8, 24, 31
Amphetamines abuse, 11
Anal
    discomfort, 47
Anemia, history of, 8, 34
Ankles
    ability to move, 58
    sprained, 60
    swollen, 39, 55
    painful, 51,
Antacids, use of, 10, 76
Antibiotics
    use of, 10
    gentamicin/streptomycin, 30
    allergy to, 52
Anticoagulants, use of, 10
Anticonvulsants, use of, 10
Anus, lesions of, 33
Anxiety, history of, 16, 56
Appetite
    loss of, 5, 16, 48, 57
    change in, 46
Arms
    weakness of, 21, 59
    motor functioning, 66, 67
    pain on movement of, 37
Arthritis, 8
Aspirin
    for pain, 26, 61
    instructions for taking, 76
Asthma, history of, 8, 9
Axilla, lumps in, 34

Back, ability to move, 58

93

Immunizations, 14
Indigestion, 46
Infection
    exposure to, 8
    upper respiratory, history of, 9,
    ear, 29
    throat, 29
    bladder, 50
    kidney, 50
Injury
    history of, 10, 29, 65
    head, 24
    eye, 28
    ear, 29
    neck, 34
    breast, 44
Insomnia, 5, 16, 57
Insulin, 65
Intercourse
    frequency of, 17
    painful, 37
Intolerance
    to certain foods, 19
    to heat or cold, 36, 56
Irritability, 20
Itch
    vaginal, 53
    scalp, 24
    with skin lesion, 23
IUD, 54

Jaundice
    history of, 12, 22
    onset of, 47
Joint
    pain, 58
    " , migratory, 51
    swelling, 61

Kidney disease/infection, history of, 40, 50
Knee
    pain in, 59
    range of motion of, 59

Labor, 55
Laceration, 78
Legs
    weakness in, 21, 59
    pain in, 38, 40, 64
    ulcers of, 40
    range of motion of, 56
Lips, cyanosis of, 38
Liver disease, 40
Loss
    of weight, 16, 43, 57

of appetite, 16, 48
of memory, 16
of hair, 24, 57
of vision, 27
of hearing, 29
of muscle strength, 31
of consciousness, 43
of urine or bowel control, 64
Lump
history and characteristics of, 34, 44, 57, 62-63
painful, 35
Lung disease, 38

Measles, 8
Memory loss, 16, 65
Menarche, age at, 53
Mental illness, history of, 8
Methadone, 12
Migraines, 26
Miscarriage, 54
Mood swings, 16
Mouth ulcers, 33
Mumps, 8
Murmur, cardiac, 39
Muscle
pulled, 60,
swollen, 61
stiff, 61
wasting, 62

Nails, cyanosis of, 38
Narcotics, 11
Nausea, 26, 31, 38, 45, 48
Neck
pain in, 25,
injury, 34
swelling, 34
lumps in, 34
Nervousness, as symptom, 16
Nipples, painful, 44
Nocturnal emission, 52
Nosebleed, 31

Odor
of sputum, 42
of urine, 49
Operation, history of, 10
Oral contraceptives, 40, 44
Orgasm, difficulty achieving, 17

Palpitations
history of, 16, 35-36
and chest pain, 38
and shortness of breath, 41
and signs of hyperthyroidism, 57

Paralysis, history of, 20, 62-63
Parasites, 48
Penicillin allergy, 11, 52
Penile discharge, 50-51
Period, menstrual 53-54, 63
Pigmentation, skin, 22
Polyps, nasal, 31
Postnasal drip, 31
Pregnancy, 45, 54
Pressure, blood
     high, 8
     medication for, 10
Prostatitis, 50
Pulse, during palpitations, 36
Purulent discharge, from penis, 50

Rash, skin, 22-24
     associated with veneral disease, 51
Respiratory infection, recent, 9
Restlessness, as symptom, 16
Rheumatic fever, history of, 8
Rhythm method, for birth control, 54
Ringing in ears, 26, 30-31

Scalp, tender, 25
Sedative drug use, 11
Seizures,history of, 64
Sexual
     functioning, 17
     intercourse, pain during, 37
Shakiness
     as symptom of hyperthyroidism, 57
     as symtom of anxiety, 16
Shortness of breath, 36, 38-41, 43
Skin
     disorders, 22-23, 25
     cyanosis of, 38
     change in color of, 44, 56
Sleep
     disturbed by pain, 6, 38, 58
     quality of, 17
     insomnia, 20
     disturbed by headache, 25,
     relieving headache, 26
     number of pillows required for, 36
     cough during, 42
Slurred speech, 65
Solvents, exposure to, 15
Sore throat/mouth, 32-33, 59
Sores, vaginal, 51
Speech, change in pattern of, 65
Spinning sensation, with vertigo,26
Spots, before eyes, 25, 27
Sprained ankle, 60
Sputum, bloody, 43

Staggering gait, 64
Stiff muscles, 61
Stillbirth, history of, 54
Stings, allergy to, 11
Stomach aches, 47
Stones, kidney, 50
Stool, 47, 48, 70
Stools, bloody, 45
Strength, loss of, 31, 62
Strep throat, 32
Streptomycin, 30
Stroke, history of, 8
Suicide, attempted, 16
Surgery, history of, 9-10
Swallowing, difficulty in, 46
Sweating
      associated with pain, 45
      with hyperthyroidism, 56
Sweats, night-time, 20
Swelling
      of neck, 34
      of ankles, 39, 55
      of legs, 40
      of muscle, joints, or bone, 61
Syphilis, 8, 51-52

Tarry stools, 47
Tenderness, of breasts, 44
Testicles, pain in, 51
Tetanus, 14
Thyroid disease, history of, 34, 56
Tightness, as headache symptom, 25
Tongue, thick or enlarged, 57
Tranquillizers, use of, 11
Tremens, delirium, 14
Tremor, 57
Tuberculosis, 8, 43

Ulcer, history of, 8,46
      of mouth, 33
      of leg, 40
Unconsciousness, history of, 10
Unsteady gait, 26, 64
Urinary frequency, 48
Urination
      pain or burning with, 48,
      nocturnal, 49
Urticaria, 9

Vagina, sores on, 33, 51
Vaginal
      itch, 53
      discharge, 53
      bleeding, 55

*RAPID LEARNING AND RETENTION THROUGH THE MEDMASTER SERIES:*

CLINICAL NEUROANATOMY MADE RIDICULOUSLY SIMPLE, by S. Goldberg
CLINICAL BIOCHEMISTRY MADE RIDICULOUSLY SIMPLE, by S. Goldberg
CLINICAL ANATOMY MADE RIDICULOUSLY SIMPLE, by S. Goldberg
CLINICAL PHYSIOLOGY MADE RIDICULOUSLY SIMPLE, by S. Goldberg
CLINICAL MICROBIOLOGY MADE RIDICULOUSLY SIMPLE, by M. Gladwin and B. Trattler
CLINICAL PHARMACOLOGY MADE RIDICULOUSLY SIMPLE, by J.M. Olson
OPHTHALMOLOGY MADE RIDICULOUSLY SIMPLE, by S. Goldberg
PSYCHIATRY MADE RIDICULOUSLY SIMPLE, by W.V. Good and J. Nelson
CLINICAL PSYCHOPHARMACOLOGY MADE RIDICULOUSLY SIMPLE, by J. Preston and J. Johnson
ACUTE RENAL INSUFFICIENCY MADE RIDICULOUSLY SIMPLE, by C. Rotellar
MEDICAL BOARDS STEP 1 MADE RIDICULOUSLY SIMPLE, by A. Carl
MEDICAL BOARDS STEP 2 MADE RIDICULOUSLY SIMPLE, by A. Carl
MEDICAL BOARDS STEP 3 MADE RIDICULOUSLY SIMPLE, by A. Carl
BEHAVIORAL MEDICINE MADE RIDICULOUSLY SIMPLE, by F. Seitz and J. Carr
USMLE BEHAVIORAL SCIENCE MADE RIDICULOUSLY SIMPLE, by F.S. Sierles
ACID-BASE, FLUIDS, AND ELECTROLYTES MADE RIDICULOUSLY SIMPLE, by R. Preston
THE FOUR-MINUTE NEUROLOGIC EXAM, by S. Goldberg
MEDICAL SPANISH MADE RIDICULOUSLY SIMPLE, by T. Espinoza-Abrams
THE DIFFICULT PATIENT, by E. Sohr
CLINICAL ANATOMY AND PATHOPHYSIOLOGY FOR THE HEALTH PROFESSIONAL, by J.V. Stewart
CONSCIOUSNESS, INFORMATION, AND MEANING: THE ORIGIN OF THE MIND, by S. Goldberg
PREPARING FOR MEDICAL PRACTICE MADE RIDICULOUSLY SIMPLE, by D.M. Lichtstein
MED'TOONS    (260 humorous medical cartoons by the author) by S. Goldberg
CLINICAL RADIOLOGY MADE RIDICULOUSLY SIMPLE, by H. Ouellette
NCLEX-RN MADE RIDICULOUSLY SIMPLE, by A. Carl
THE PRACTITIONER'S POCKET PAL: ULTRA RAPID MEDICAL REFERENCE, by J. Hancock
NEUROLOGIC LOCALIZATION (MacIntosh computer program), by S. Goldberg

Try your bookstore. For further information and ordering send for the MedMaster catalog at MedMaster, P.O. Box 640028, Miami FL 33164. Or see http://www.medmaster.net for current information. Email: mmbks@aol.com